DATE DUE

June 5, 09	
Oct 12, 2009	
March 26, 2010	
Aug 5, 2010	
DEC 19 2011	
Jan 20, 2012	
Oct 26, 2013	
April 2, 2014	
July 23, 2014	
Sept 10, 2014	
Nov 26, 2014	
Feb 1, 2016	
Jan 11, 2017	

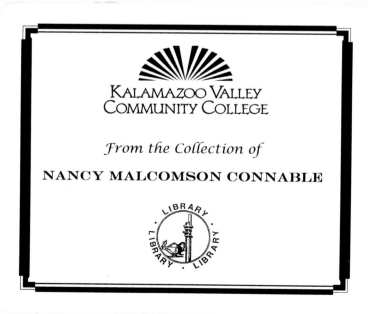

YOU ARE WHAT YOU ATE

An Rx for the Resistant Diseases
of the 21st Century

by Sherry A. Rogers, M.D., F.A.C.A.I., F.A.A.E.M.
F.A.A.F.P.

1988

Prestige Publishing
Box 3068, 3502 Brewerton Road
Syracuse, NY 13220

For information address Prestige Publishers,
Box 3161, 3502 Brewerton Road, Syracuse, N.Y. 13220

Library of Congress Catalog Card Number: 88-090874

ISBN 0-9618821-1-5

Printed in the United States.

YOU ARE WHAT YOU ATE

Table of Contents

Dedication

Disclaimer

Acknowledgments

Foreword

Sherry A. Rogers, M.D., F.A.C.A.I., F.A.A.E.M.,
                F.A.A.F.P.
Northeast Center for Environmental Medicine
2800 West Genesee Street
Syracuse, NY 13219

1988

Dedication

To Rob, my most precious gift from God, who nearly starved to death while discovering that he hates macrobiotic food. Eighteen years ago when we were bride and groom, little did I suspect that a love so strong could grow even more wonderful through the years. Nor did I ever dream that in addition to this indescribable blessing, my groom would continually nourish and groom me into all that I was capable of being.

And to our staff, in particular Barbara Mulvana, Shirley Gallinger, Carol Fenton, and Frank Mulvana, who over many years, through computer crashes and hectic days have worked diligently to help patients learn and grow along with us in our quest for health.

Disclaimer

This work is a guide for people who are working in concert with a certified health professional. It is in no way meant to be a prescription for anyone attempting to heal themselves without medical monitoring and guidance.

Acknowledgements

Thank you Jackie Roshia for your tireless typing and editorial assistance.

CHAPTER I

INTRODUCTION

WHO CARRIES THE BALL?

Do you want to get well?

Do you want to awaken after five hours of
sleep playful, laughing and
enthusiastic to tackle the day?

Do you want to reach new levels of wellness,
physically and mentally?

Then you have chosen "educate". For in the
world of medicine there are only two choices:

TO MEDICATE OR EDUCATE

If you prefer to medicate, you choose
conventional medicine where symptoms are given an
accepted term or name (diagnosis). Then blood
tests and x-rays are done to confirm that the
accepted term has been correctly applied to this
conglomeration of symptoms. After that, it's
merely a matter of trial and error to determine
which drug will relieve all the symptoms. If
success is not imminent, surgery is considered.
Next case.

For example - Mr. Jones complains of a
headache.

Through the diagnostic process he has a
chemical profile and CAT scan.

He receives a magic label:
"Mr. Jones, you have migraines".

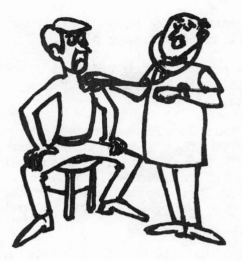

To medicate

or

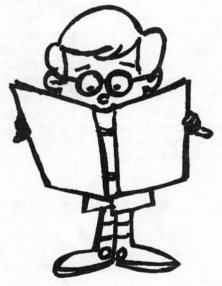

educate ------

That is the question.

He gets his treatment: a prescription for
pain pills and migraine pills.

Mr. Jones goes home to watch T.V. and drinks
beer and eats chocolate and has a
migraine.

What's wrong? Mr. Jones has chosen a doctor
who does not search for a cause of symptoms. He
merely medicates. He thinks a headache is a
codeine deficiency. Furthermore, he has given the
unspoken message to Mr. Jones: eat, drink, and
breathe whatever you want. I have a pill for
everything.

On the other hand, if Mr. Jones wants to take
an active part in his health and find the causes
for his symptoms and get rid of them without
medication, this requires work. He must be
educated. This takes time and insurance companies
don't pay for time spent in educating patients.
Also, Mr. Jones will have to seek out a physician
trained in finding causes and interested in
educating the patient. And he has to learn to
listen to his body—not just when it belts him
between the eyes, but when it whispers in his ear.
And Mr. Jones will have to modify his lifestyle.
He will have to read that boring book,
The E.I. Syndrome.

But he has a choice: To medicate or educate.

And the choice extends far beyond the present
illness. It extends to his day to day well being
and his overall life span. For the decision he
makes today will have an effect on all his other
symptoms and even his future decision-making
process itself.

So the very first thing Mr. Jones has to
decide is to whom will he give responsibility

for his health?   His doctor or himself? Who is going to carry the ball?

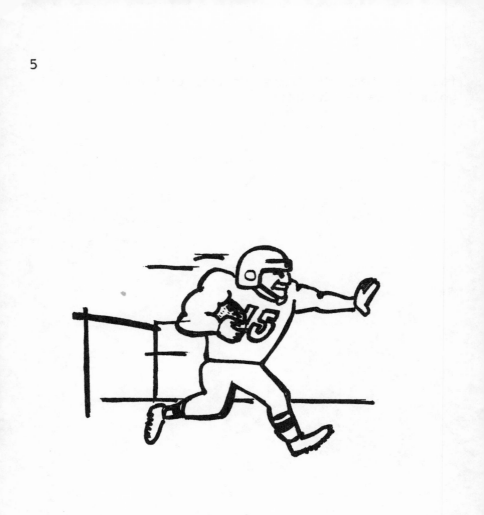

And who is going to carry the ball for your
health?

Your doctor is your coach or consultant. You
are the player who decides whether the game is won.
Don't make the coach carry the ball. No one ever
won that way.

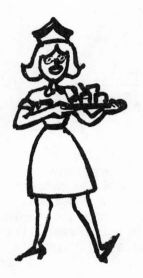

Every medicine has its side effects and drawbacks and merely masks symptoms.

Many people take extra drugs to cover the side effects of their primary drugs.

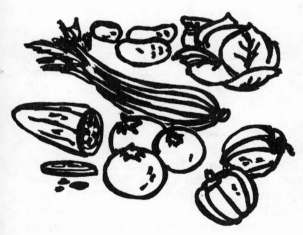

Every medicine puts an extra stress on the body's detoxification system.

Why not have your food be your medicine while first strengthening your detox system with appropriate nutrients?

CHAPTER II

E.I. IN A NUTSHELL

E.I., or environmental illness, can masquerade as many common medical symptoms and diseases: migraines, chronic exhaustion, recurrent infection, chronic post nasal drip, asthma, bronchitis, irritable bowel, colitis, spastic colon, chronic cystitis, traumatic arthritis, vasculitis, sarcoid, lupus, eczema, psoriasis, Sjogren's syndrome, depression, spaciness, inability to concentrate, hyperactivity, violent mood swings, urethritis, prostatitis, TMJ (temporo-mandibular joint), chronic EBV (Epstein Barr Virus), rheumatoid arthritis, degenerative arthritis, neuritis, endometriosis, dizziness, chronic Candida, chemical hypersensitivity, infertility, poor memory, panic attacks, weakness and many undiagnosable maladies. For more information, consult our 650 page book, The E.I. Syndrome (Prestige Publishing, Box 3161, 3502 Brewerton Rd., Syracuse, NY 13220, $15 and $3 postage and handling).

The ecologic approach to health has brought health answers and wellness to people who never thought they could be free of symptoms again. And I was one of these people.

However, in a small percentage of people, the ecologic approach is not enough. There is a small group for whom nothing has helped. There is another much larger group who are 50 to 95% improved, but they have not achieved that 100% that they know they could have. We've discovered further alternatives that are available for those who know that clean food and water, rotation diets, good environmental controls for pollens, dusts, molds and chemicals, correction of nutritional

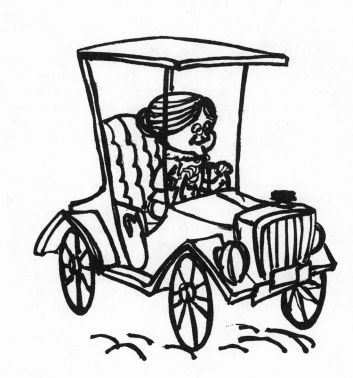

Age has nothing to do with fatigue and
exhaustion. That is one of medicine's many cop-outs
or myths.

deficiencies, reduction of stress and hyposensitizing injections are not quite enough.

For these people, their bodies are still not unloaded enough, in spite of having worked through the total load, to allow them to heal. Some of them are so sensitive, they cannot even come out of their homes; they react to every chemical that abounds in the world outside of their bedrooms or an environmental unit. With the thousands of cases that have been observed during the practice of environmental medicine, we have seen one astounding fact; the body can heal just about anything, if given the opportunity. So what has arrested healing for these people?

For some, they have neglected to reduce their chemical environment sufficiently to allow healing. They still live with gas appliances or wood stoves, carpets, eat processed foods or work under very adverse conditions.

But for some people that last part of the total load seems to be far too illusive, it seems to have escaped their grasp; that is until now.

You'll recall in The E.I. Syndrome how diagnoses of sarcoidosis, lupus, multiple sclerosis, intractable cardiac arrhythmia, schizophrenia, ulcerative colitis, degenerative, traumatic, osteo and rheumatoid arthritides and a multitude of other end-of-the-road conditions were either totally cleared or remarkably improved. Those people lovingly taught me that I should never stop looking for solutions, regardless of how narrowly I viewed a prognosis.

When we closely evaluate why some people are not better, it's obvious: they are just plain not sick enough to do all that is necessary. And that's alright. They have been educated and have chosen their paths. We all have a certain time when we choose to make time to coordinate a health program. The missing part of the total load boat varies from person to person. But here's a quick checklist to be sure you have done all you can up to this point to heal your environmental illness or E.I. And bear in mind E.I. really encompasses every chronic disease, chronic Candida, and those nebulous chronic symptoms of unwellness that do not yet merit a name by the current medical system. In the following total load synopsis, obviously not everyone needs everything that is listed. But you should persist until you are free of symptoms. And if symptoms still persist, then the remainder of this book is for you.

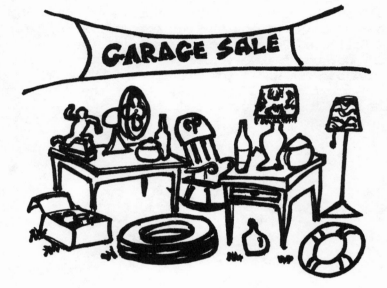

Get rid of as much junk as possible from your home, especially the bedroom oasis. Why have things outgasing and collecting dust that you will never use?

E.I. Checklist

Is your inhalant load covered?

_____ (1) Have you exposed mold plates in the bedroom and other places you most commonly frequent? If the mold is high, have you recultured until the plates show your environmental controls are good? (Anyone can send for petri dishes or mold plates to expose in the home. Directions are included plus a return mailer. A list of the types and numbers of molds identified by a Ph.D. mycologist will be mailed to you as soon as the last mold has stopped growing. This is usually within 2-7 weeks. Petri dishes or mold plates, as they are called, are available from Mold Survey Service, 2800 W. Genesee St Syracuse, NY 13219, $15 each).

_____ (2) Is there an air cleaner in the bedroom, regularly serviced?

_____ (3) Is the carpet out of the bedroom?

_____ (4) Is there an air conditioner in the bedroom?

_____ (5) Has there been removal of all objects except the bed if you are very sensitive (especially bureaus and closet contents)?

_____ (6) Has there been cutting of nearby trees, installing gutters, trenches, and dry wells about the house to reduce dampness; correction of leaks, removal of old wallpaper, bathroom tiles and other hidden sources of mold?

_____ (7) Test titrated inhalants (pollens, dust, molds, mites) and receive injections twice weekly until symptoms are clear. Return to twice weekly interval if symptoms recur.

_____ (8) Break down mixes (trees, grasses, molds) and test to individual components of mixes that are especially allergenic.

_____ (9) Test newer molds.

_____ (10) Retest phenol and glycerine if injections cause a problem.

_____ (11) Do you have cotton mattress covers and bedding, regularly washed? Did you evaluate an old foil covered mattress?

_____ (12) Is there regular wet dusting to remove and not merely redistribute the dust?

_____ (13) Did you remove allergenic animals?

Has food allergy been ruled out?

_____ (1) Use glass bottled spring water for a one month trial.

_____ (2) Did you evaluate the rare food, rotated diet for one month?

_____ (3) If there was no difference, a different rare food diet, not necessarily rotated of extremely rare foods and as organic as possible should be evaluated on the chance that your initial one contained hidden food allergies.

_____ (4) Have you fasted five days?

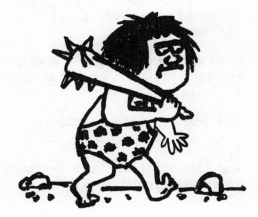

The caveman diet or rare food diet is a must for anyone who doesn't feel wonderful. Hidden food allergies are extremely common.

_____ (5) Did you evaluate food testing and daily injections for at least 6 months?

Is Candida a problem?

_____ (1) Did you do a ferment-free (bread, cheese, alcohol, vinegar, catsup, mayonnaise, salad dressing, packaged foods) and sugar-free (anything with corn syrup, maple syrup, cane sugar, dextrose, maltose, malt, honey) diet for two months,

_____ (2) with a known reputable source of acidophilus such as Vital Dophilus used for 6 months?

_____ (3) Did you evaluate a trial of Nystatin with all of the above for 2 months?

_____ (4) and the addition of a 2-4 week trial of ketoconazole (Nizoral)?

Is there a hidden nutritional deficiency?

_____ (1) Have all the latest vitamin and mineral assays been drawn? There are new tests available every few months, that we didn't have before.

_____ (2) Have special tests for amino acids and essential fatty acids been drawn?

_____ (3) Correct deficiencies then re-assess the balance.

_____ (4) Make a special appointment to assess biochemical nutritional status and diet quality.

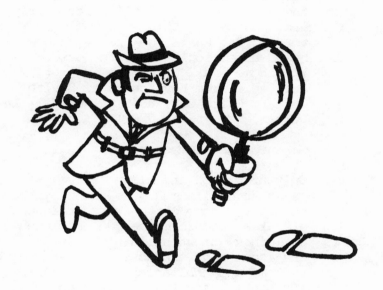

In your search for wellness, follow methodically the ecologic checklist for clues of areas you have missed. Reread The E.I. Syndrome.

The toughest problem: the chemical environment

_____ (1) Create an oasis (preferably bedroom) where you can clear.

_____ (2) If you can't clear, stay outdoors in a safe area like near the ocean or go to the Dallas environmental unit. (If you are considering this, you would be wise to read Dr. Rea's book first on how to build an ecologically safe house. Your Home and Your Health is available from Environmental Health Center, Suite 200, 8345 Walnut Hill Ln Dallas, TX 75231, $20.)

_____ (3) Go on oxygen temporarily.

_____ (4) Only after you are clear can you re-enter environments to identify the culprits. Some of the worst triggers are urea foam formaldehyde insulated buildings, tight buildings, traffic and industrial exhausts, gas heating systems and appliances, glues and adhesives (carpet, tiles, cupboards, furnishings), gasoline (benzene) and oils (pumps, furnaces, machines), plastics and synthetic materials (xylene, formaldehyde, toluene, acrylics, vinyls, benzene, phenol), cleaning solutions and air fresheners (xylene, benzene, trichloroethylene, phenol), pesticides, and municipal water (chlorine, chloroform).

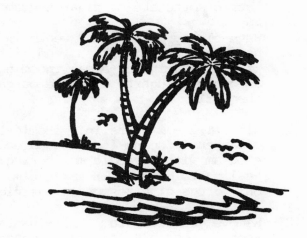

You need a home oasis, usually the bedroom. If you can't awaken feeling great, where are you going the rest of the day?

_____ (5) Chemically-free personal grooming is mandatory: no scented cosmetics, deodorants, mousses, shampoos, soaps, lotions, sprays, astringents, conditioners, new fabrics, polyester or acrylic, dry cleaned items, detergents, fabric softeners or cigarette smoke.

_____ (6) Have plenty of fans and vents in the home and office: fresh (and filtered if in contaminated area) incoming air, adequate enough to displace outgassed chemicals

_____ (7) Allow 1/2 - 2 years in a chemically clean environment (on a sound ecologic program with periodic monitoring) for healing to occur. It takes time. Only drugs give responses overnight.

_____ (8) Remove yourself from contaminants as soon as possible, shower, cleanse the bowel, take anti-oxidants and recover as quickly as possible.

_____ (9) Do you need to test chemicals? (We published the protocol in the National Institutes of Health medical journal, Environmental Health Perspectives, volume 76, pp 195-198, 1987.)

_____ (10) Do you need a detoxification program?

_____ (11) Have you reread The E.I. Syndrome?

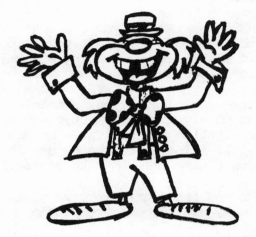

A sense of humor has long been known as a stimulant to the immune system. If you don't have a healthy one, get some professional counseling to see what holds you back.

IS YOUR BRAIN IN A HEALING MODE?

_____ (1) Do you need to be ill? Are you more comfortable being ill than well? If so, you need a professional counselor.

_____ (2) Do you practice positive imagery and not just wishful thinking?

_____ (3) Have you reduced your personal stress to show your body that you respect and love it? Are you making a commitment to lifestyle changes and wellness?

_____ (4) Have you changed your schedule to purposely make time for exercise, meditation and healing? Or are you still clinging to the excuse that you don't have time to make yourself well?

_____ (5) Do you frequently involve yourself with "up", happy, positive people?

_____ (6) Do you make sure you sing and laugh several times a day?

_____ (7) Do you set realistic goals and periodically assess your progress?

_____ (8) Do you feel optimistic and believe you are worth the effort, and that you will get well?

Have you ruled out special problems? For
example:

_____ (1)   the need to have another thorough
            medical exam?

_____ (2)   test hormones or neurotransmitters

_____ (3)   test ionization and electromagnetic
            field effects

_____ (4)   a non-supportive spouse

_____ (5)   consider phenolics.

Note: The above areas (2,3,5) are so new your only
       recourse will be to see the doctor for an
       explanation of these. They are not written
       up yet.

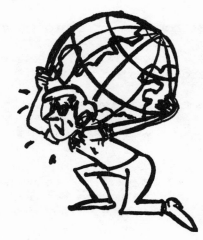

Everyone has problems. But some people don't choose to lessen their burdens in order to allow healing to proceed. Try to level with yourself or get professional help.

HEALING CANCERS

In searching for a clue to see why a small sector of people afflicted with environmental illness could not attain total recovery, I started looking at cancer patients. I discovered that there were people who had healed cancers that were termed incurable. For example, Dr. Anthony Sattilaro, (his book Recalled by Life, Avon Books, a division of Hearst Corporation, 1970 Broadway, New York, NY 10019, 1984) is a physician in his mid forties who had cancer of the prostate, which metastasized to the skull. He was given a maximum of three to six months to live by all of his colleagues who were specialists in various aspects of his treatment. As a director of a Philadelphia hospital, he had access to everything that medicine could offer. As a last resort, he went on a macrobiotic program and totally cleared his cancer and his metastasis and is alive and well.

Elaine Nussbaum (her book Recovery, Japan Publications, Kodansha International, Ltd. through Harper and Row Publishers, 10 East 53rd Street, New York, NY 10022, 1986), is a young mother in her thirties who developed cancer of the ovaries. This was, needless to say, the biggest shock of her life, but she geared up for it and ate as healthfully as possible, did everything she could with positive imagery and had a wonderful family support system behind her. In spite of all this, she continued to decline, as she had radiation treatments and chemotherapy. She was weakened, nauseated and bald. Eventually her ovarian cancer spread to her lungs and liver and even the vertebral bodies of her back bone. The metastatic cancer caused her spine to collapse and left her in a wheelchair, hairless, withered, ridden with pain and incapacitated. She, likewise, wrote about her victory over cancer with the macrobiotic approach and has dissolved all of her cancer, and its metastases; her bones are healed and she is a practicing counselor this day.

When I read about these two cases, I figured, "Heck, if they can cure cancer, then E.I. ought to be a piece of cake". But I couldn't understand why it should be so beneficial, until I started researching the macrobiotic approach. Still there appeared to be so many drawbacks to macrobiotics that I put this information on the back shelf and pursued detoxification as the route to wellness.

CHAPTER III

NUTRITION: DO YOU HAVE THE VULNERABILITY FACTOR?

DON'T TOUCH THOSE VITAMINS

It's no secret that many myopic members of the medical profession are on a warpath against vitamins and recommend that lay people do not take them. In fact, they go so far as to state that the American diet provides all the nutrition that the average person needs. I made a search of the literature myself, to find that there are scores of papers proving marked mineral and vitamin deficiencies in many countries, including our own, and extending to all ages of our population. Here is just a minute sample regarding one of scores of nutrients, zinc.

Elsborg in a study of 403 elderly Danes residing in their own homes showed that zinc intake was low in 87% of the people. Holden showed that 68% of 22 American men and women eating self-selected diets were found to consume less than two-thirds of the RDA of zinc, while Hambridge showed that pregnant women ingested only about two-thirds of the recommended daily dietary allowance. The studies go on and on.

Most likely the same physicians and dieticians who recommend no vitamins are also the ones who make biochemical blunders daily by recommending hydrogenated grocery store corn oils and margarines for those with elevated cholesterols, thereby increasing their intakes of trans fatty acids, which actually stress the body chemistry and accelerate degenerative diseases (see the <u>E.I. Syndrome</u>). This same mindset supports the ingestion of

processed foods which contain inferior levels of
vitamins E, B6, and minerals like zinc and
magnesium. These deficiencies coupled with the
trans fatty acids push degeneration or deterioration
(aging) even faster.

We did a study of over 400 people who
consecutively reported to our office for diagnosis
and management of allergic and environmentally
induced illnesses (E.I.), and over 50 percent of
these people had a zinc deficiency. Over a third
of the others who were not deficient were
marginally just above the lowest level of normal.

Upon studying the comments made by doctors
opposed to nutritional supplementation, I finally
figured out how physicians can confidently assert
that vitamins are not needed.

1. They do not study the biochemistry
   literature to learn of the astounding flood
   of evidence for supplementation for a
   variety of conditions, and they do
   not seek out the literature to learn that
   their claims of nutritional adequacy are
   not substantiated; nor do they initiate
   their own studies. In other words,
   ignorance is bliss.

2. They don't realize that symptoms of
   nutritional deficiencies are subtle.
   Medicine is excellent at diagnosing endstage
   diseases such as diabetes or hepatitis where
   grossly abnormal functions of blood tests
   occur. However, long before blood test
   abnormalities present themselves, people
   have symptoms. It's the early warning
   symptoms like chronic tiredness that alert
   one to find a cause before end-stage organ
   failure occurs. Unfortunately tests, like
   the chemical profile that is drawn as part
   of an annual physical examination, are not
   sensitive enough to show abnormalities
   at the early stage of disease. Therefore,

absence of blood test abnormality is
assumed to mean absence of disease; an
absolutely erroneous assumption.

Medicine goes one step further labeling
people who complain of these early symptoms
as hypochondriacs, whereas in reality there
is no such thing as a hypochondriac. If a
person complains of something, even if it is
all in his head, it's the job of a physician
to find out why he is complaining and try to
help him. Therefore, no complaint is
without merit, nor should it be ignored.

3. Oftentimes, physicians are put off by the
claims of individuals recovering from
vitamin deficiencies. In other words,
they'll hear that vitamin B6 cleared one
person's PMS, another person's depression,
another person's fatigue, and another
person's carpal tunnel syndrome. So they
erroneously assume, having just graduated
from the school of cookbook medicine, that
B6 deficiency can't cause any of those
symptoms. In essence, however, B6 is
crucial in over 30 enzyme systems and not
everyone, because of biochemical
individuality, shorts the same enzymes.
Therefore, different symptoms can occur.
Zinc, for example, is crucial in over 90
enzymes. One person may short enzymes
1-5, another may short enzymes 50-55, and
another may short another set of enzymes.
They will, clearly, all have totally
different symptoms.

And we can't blame the current state of the
art entirely, for the patient shares some
of the burden. Many people with nutritional
deficiencies, because they have occurred so
slowly don't appreciate how bad they really
feel. They have become used to feeling
below par as a way of life. When an astute
physician elicits minor symptoms, then hunts

for, finds, and corrects the causative deficiency, the patient experiences for the first time in years what feeling good is really all about. If you haven't felt good for many years, you tend to make many rationalizations and assume it's just part of stress or getting older. But as many people have told us, after their nutritional deficiencies were corrected, they haven't felt so good in years. And in some cases, they have never felt so good, ever before.

Others have learned to ignore or tune-out early warning symptoms because they fear being labeled hypochondriacs. Because we operate with a medical system that is not designed to diagnose and treat early body malfunction, we as physicians tend to label people as hypochondriacs and crocks when we can't find a cause for their complaints. This helps us save face.

4. Physicians fail to consider that just because the blood level for a nutrient falls within the "normal range", that this may not necessarily mean that this is the normal level for this particular person.

There is a vast difference between normal and optimal. Many of the values derived for nutritional supplements are drawn from a number of people who are not necessarily optimally healthy or feeling their best. For example, the normal level of B12 is 200-900. That's a tremendous range when you realize other levels, such as thyroid are much smaller. This suggests that many of the people at the lower end of the scale were not at optimal health, and it also suggests that if the range of normal is so

huge, then how do we know that one
particular individual's best level of
function isn't 900 or even more, say 1200?

5. Opponents of vitamins argue that many of the
vitamins are toxic and dangerous. This is
true, but so is everything in the world
toxic or dangerous at some particular dose,
including air and water. Everything has a
bell-shaped curve of maximum desired effect.

But with a knowledge of human biochemistry
and periodic monitoring of levels, how
dangerous can a program be? Proclaiming
danger is merely a way of covering up for
lack of knowledge. Wouldn't it be more
honest to simply refer to a specialist who
does have special knowledge in nutritional
biochemistry instead of denying the
existence of untested deficiencies? That
would be like me saying that no one needs a
brain surgeon, since I don't know anything
about doing brain surgery.

Likewise, there is a tremendous difference
between corrective levels and maintenance levels.
Corrective levels are necessarily unbalanced to
balance or correct an imbalance (the deficiency) in
a person's chemistry. Then, after a few months,
when the correction has been made and monitored, a
maintenance dosage can be employed, which is much
lower and is, of necessity, a much more balanced
scheme of nutrients.

For example, in correcting over 500 patients
with abnormally low levels of RBC zinc, I was
amazed to find that 2 and 3 times the RDA of 15
mg/day of zinc did not correct many people over a
period of two months. Many required levels of 90
mg. or over. This is potentially dangerous because
such extremely high levels can lower copper,
molybdenum and manganese.

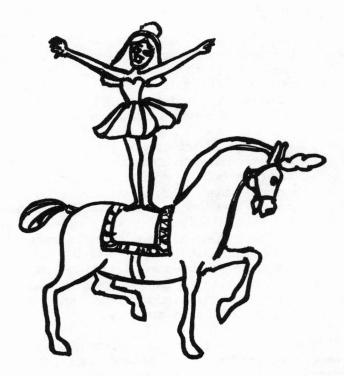

Correcting a nutritional deficiency requires quite a balancing act. Some physicians do not have the biochemical knowledge to do it. For example, they would not know that incorrectly correcting your zinc can cause deficiencies in copper, magnesium, manganese, molybdenum, and more.

I, for one, was a conventionally trained physician who, for years, suffered exhaustion for no reason and kept looking through all of my medical textbooks to try to find a reason. One of the final answers was that I had multiple nutritional deficiencies, many of which could not be corrected until I had identified further hidden nutritional deficiencies.

For example, my vitamin A level was extremely low (I had eczema, so I probably used it up prematurely. The result of a vitamin A deficiency is poor mucosal barrier integrity, which in turn made me more vulnerable to Candida). Anyway, after large doses of vitamin A, my level was not corrected. It wasn't until I found that I was zinc deficient that I could correct my vitamin A level. For you see, zinc is crucial in the enzyme alcohol dehydrogenase, which converts the primary form of vitamin A as retinol, into the first metabolic breakdown step or retinaldehyde. Without sufficient levels of the zinc dependent enzyme alcohol dehydrogenase, I could take vitamin A until I grew gills and it would not raise my level. And if I had measured the wrong test, a serum zinc instead of an RBC or erythrocyte zinc, I would not have found the zinc deficiency at all. Likewise even intravenous magnesium administration wouldn't correct my erythrocyte magnesium deficiency which manifested itself as months of intolerable back spasm in an area of old injury, until I had discovered and corrected my manganese deficiency.

So you see, not only is the field of nutrition complex, but one undetected deficiency can lead to another, which in turn leads to increased vulnerability for various disease states. In other words, it snowballs or spreads.

This domino effect of one deficiency leading to another, most likely contributes to the spreading phenomenon of E.I. The spreading phenomenon occurs when the victim starts reacting to more and more things that never bothered him before. The mechanism is partly due to an accumulation or backlog of chemicals being presented to a nutritionally incomplete detoxification system.

This completely baffles the physician untrained in nutritional biochemistry and environmental medicine because what he sees is a person with over a dozen vague complaints of exhaustion, feeling "unreal" or spacey and depressed for no reason. These patients also have a half dozen recognizable complaints like migraines, chronic sinusitis, spastic colon, arthralgia, or asthma.

On top of this, all the exams, x-rays, and blood tests are normal. And to make matters worse, as the patient snowballs further, he starts reacting to things that never before bothered him ---various foods, stores, cigarette smoke, cleansers, construction glues, new carpets and more.

Then the last straw comes when the spreading phenomenon has reached its peak and he reacts faster and more vigorously to these triggers. By this time, everyone, including the patient is left doubting the sanity of the patient; and only because modern medicine is not well-versed in the molecular biology and biochemistry of the spreading phenomenon.

A typical scenario is a young woman who gets hooked on sweets, colas and processed foods. She gets married, starts taking the birth control pill and smoking. As she gets more depleted of nutrients, she gets colds more easily and is put on antibiotics. As she feels more drained, she has

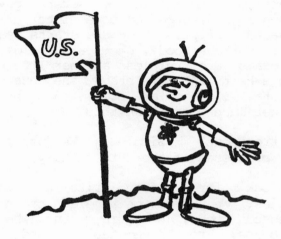

If we can put a man on the moon, it seems that we should routinely look at his vitamin and mineral levels.

more coffee and sweets in attempt to increase her energy. Then she gets recurrent vaginal infections and starts with intestinal symptoms of gas, bloating and indigestion. Her childhood hay-fever symptoms of chronic headaches, and postnasal drip resurface and she slowly descends to constant tiredness and unwarranted depression. She may have a pregnancy, root canal, auto accident, severe psychological stress such as a divorce, or move into a new house or renovated office. Soon she starts reacting with symptoms to various foods, chemicals, molds, but all medical exams are fruitless and her life seems to be coming to a halt. At this stage she has full-blown environmental illness or E.I., that believe it or not, can get much worse than this.

The treatment? Simple. We just reverse the unhealthy processes of the 20th century.

We look for hidden vitamin and mineral deficiencies. We put her on a diet of no sweets, no processed foods, heavy in greens, whole grains, seeds, beans, root vegetables and sometimes mineral-rich seaweeds. We treat the Candida problem. We test her for hidden mold sensitivities and treat them. It's a rare victim who isn't loaded with them. We have her adopt a chemically less-contaminated lifestyle by getting rid of smelly cleansers, fragrant cosmetics and toiletries, old carpets, use air purification devices and more. Later we can test for hidden food and chemical sensitivities if needed.

In essence, we whittle away at her total 20th century body burden or load (as we described in The E.I. Syndrome), until she is unloaded enough to heal and feel better than she has ever remembered.

Most likely, in years to come, medicine will no longer rely on such gross tests of end organ failure as the chemical profile, such as it exists today. Most likely, we will draw a few tubes of blood and be able to assay within minutes your every vitamin, mineral, essential fatty acid, and amino acid. Until that time, we have to continue doing blood assays as money (insurance companies seem to harbor a particular disdain for nutrient levels) and availability of specific tests permit. A few pieces of the puzzle are far better than no pieces at all.

ARE YOU A NUTRITIONAL TIME BOMB WAITING TO GO OFF?

When every doctor has been stumped, after all the blood tests and x-rays come back negative and yet still you are caught in a maze of seemingly unrelated symptoms, even you will begin to doubt your own sanity. Most likely you have the vulnerability factor: an unrecognized nutritional deficiency.

Everyone was excited about the face-lift that the office was getting. New pastel paints were chosen, a lovely beige carpet was glued down, new draperies and chairs and artificial potted plants were added. It was about time that the old office had some renovations. As the work continued, however, one person became progressively sicker.

Gina at first started having headaches, then she found she couldn't concentrate. She was depressed for no reason. When she got home in the evening she was so exhausted she could think of nothing except going straight to bed. Slowly other symptoms started. Every time she ate chocolate she would have a severe headache. This had never happened before.

Every time she went back into the building she could smell the glues and the paints and the new carpet. She asked her co-workers if it bothered them, but everybody just looked at her as though she were a little strange. She went to her doctor's finally to have a good physical and he gave her a clean bill of health.

After a while she started getting extremely nauseated; she just could no longer concentrate. She went to several other doctors and again was told that everything was fine. With time she began to doubt her own sanity, for after all, everyone else was happy in the new office and she was the only one reacting. If there were something in there, surely other people would be involved. And if there were something wrong with her, surely one of the six physicians that she eventually saw would have found it. The reason they didn't however, is that Gina is one of the thousands of people who have E.I. or Environmental Illness. And out of over half a million physicians in the United States there are less than 400 trained physicians who have passed the oral and written examinations of the American Academy of Environmental Medicine, and who are trained in diagnosing and treating environmental illness.

One of the first things we found in Gina's blood workup was that her red blood cell (RBC) zinc was abnormally low. This is most likely one of the factors that made her so vulnerable. For when the zinc becomes low, the body is not able to detoxify chemicals as quickly. Zinc is crucial in over a dozen pathways in the detoxification mechanism of the liver. Normally the liver is constantly at work detoxifying the chemicals that are in food, air and water. But when a zinc deficiency is present, one major detoxification enzyme, alcohol dehydrogenase, can suffer. This is the primary enzyme for the breakdown (or detoxication or biotransformation) of many chemicals.

When this enzyme is no longer functional, the chemicals must find a different pathway to follow. Take trichloroethylene, which is in many people's blood streams from the dry cleaning fluid in their clothes and carpets, glues and construction adhesives at home and at work, as well as in the drinking water in most municipalities as an industrial contaminant. It's also used to decaffeinate coffee. As a prevalent solvent, it's widespread in its use in the United States.

Chemicals can enter the blood through the lungs. All things that you breathe or smell can get into the blood and brain. In the blood they get to take a pass through the liver, since this is one of nature's check points to help keep us clear of poisons and toxins. Once they enter the liver to be detoxified, there isn't just one pathway, but sometimes as much as a dozen different routes a chemical can take. The route that is taken depends on which route is available and which ones are already taken and busy detoxifying other chemicals that got there first.

When the alcohol dehydrogenase pathway is blocked, as in a zinc deficiency, one of the breakdown or detox pathways a chemical can take leads to the formation of chloral hydrate. You may remember this name as the old "Mickey Finn" or knock-out drops, which cause exactly the same symptoms that people with environmental illness experience: tremendous exhaustion, dizziness, nausea, inability to concentrate, spaciness, numbness and tingling in the extremities, mood swings and much more.

Detoxification pathways can be weakened in two ways. They can be overloaded by too many other chemicals or they can be improperly functioning due to nutrient deficiencies. When this happens, chemicals that before never bothered a person, now start giving him symptoms. He can no longer tolerate cigarette smoke, or perfumes or certain stores, or the smell of certain cleansers and he can have headaches or dizziness or nausea or cough triggered by each exposure.

When the detoxification system is ailing, (from chemical exposure overload and/or nutrient deficiencies), subsequent chemicals from daily exposures get backed up in the blood. Without enough enzymes or chemical pathways available to accommodate them, chemical exposures that never before bothered someone will now cause alarming reactions that seem out of proportion or distorted.

To compound the problem the responses are not consistent from one exposure time to the next due to many factors: (1) shifting of pathway availability as the body attempts to cope with the overload, and (2) the total body burden which is never the same any two moments in time. To the observer, it really looks like the person reacting is a hypochondriac. And the bewildered reactor is left not even able to think rationally, much less figure out what is happening.

For example the morning you have coffee and a donut for breakfast and get caught in heavy traffic, may be the day that you get a headache and mood swings from the newly glued baseboard molding in the office. Whereas on a day when you have spent the weekend in fresh air and had a healthful breakfast, the glue doesn't bother you.

With a build up of chemicals in the blood, cell membranes are attacked and become weak. Chemicals enter the cell easily and damage further regulatory chemistry. The brain membranes and cells are particularly vulnerable. Also, the ubiquitous mitochondrial membranes which are responsible for energy synthesis are easily damaged. So inability to concentrate and exhaustion mysteriously emerge.

So Let's See What Damage a Deficiency In Just One Nutrient Can Do

An undiscovered zinc deficiency can lead to poor absorption and metabolism of other nutrients. For example zinc is of primary importance in an enzyme called carbonic anhydrase, which is responsible for making the hydrochloric acid or HCL which is crucial for absorption of minerals. Alcohol dehydrogenase is a zinc dependent enzyme necessary for the absorption of vitamin A. You can take vitamin A in extremely high doses and never clear a deficiency of it, if you do not have proper alcohol dehydrogenase enzyme to convert vitamin A from retinol to retinaldehyde, its first breakdown step.

Finding one nutritional deficiency is a clue that there are others. It's very unlikely that a person can develop a singular biochemical deficiency.

Pyridoxine kinase is an important zinc enzyme, which facilitates the breakdown of vitamin B6 to its first usable step, pyridoxal-5-phosphate. This goes on to be necessary in the synthesis of all brain neurotransmitters or chemicals that are responsible for our moods. You can begin to see how a deficiency of one single mineral can spread into a maze of symptoms which confuse the physician untrained in environmental medicine.

Zinc enzymes are necessary for proper insulin storage. Does this relate to the high incidence of hypoglycemia symptoms seen in E.I.? Zinc is crucial in DNA polymerase, an enzyme that keeps our genetics stable. Does this explain why after a particular chemical exposure we were suddenly different, never to return to totally normal non-sensitive beings again? Dr. Barbara McClintock received the Nobel Prize (1983) thirty years after she discovered that genes can change in response to an organism's attempt to adapt to a foreign environment. Without proper enzymes to control the "jumping genes" as they are called, they are more prone to distortion or re-arrangement. The result can be a new program: that of the monster called E.I.

Zinc and taurine form a conjugate that protects cell membranes. Is this why people with E.I. are prone to fluid retention, crazy mood swings (brain swelling), exhaustion, cardiac arrhythmias (when it feels like your heart is doing cartwheels), and chemical sensitivity? It's highly likely since these are all phenomena of sick or defective membranes. With deficient zinc, the cell membranes are left naked or vulnerable to attack by chemicals. (And more chemicals are spilling over into the blood because the liver is less able to handle them when it's zinc-dependent detoxification enzymes are suffering). When chemicals attack membranes, they develop holes and leaks. The cell behaves abnormally and the symptoms are determined by which organs' cells suffer the most.

If brain cells are leaky, you get all the crazy mental symptoms, spacey, etc. If it's heart cells, you get palpitations, if it's blood vessel cells, you get swelling or vasculitis. If it's liver mitochondrial walls, you have poor energy.

Many types of saran type plastics (vinylidene chlorides) are metabolized into aldehydes, as are many rubber products. Candida toxicity can also produce aldehydes, as do many environmental pollutants, such as exhaust fumes and formaldehyde from myriads of home and office furnishings. These aldehydes can mimic some of the tremendous brain fog, or inability to concentrate, exhaustion, poor memory and dizziness so classic in chemically intolerant people. They can also proceed to contribute to the chemistry that produces cancer years later. Carbonic anhydrase is a zinc dependent enzyme which has to do with buffering of this acetaldehyde and metabolizing it. Obviously if zinc is deficient in this enzyme, there is reason for further accentuation of the severe depression and brain fog, which is so commonly seen in victims of E.I.

So what am I saying? If zinc is deficient in just one enzyme, carbonic anhydrase, the body can start reacting to Candida, exhaust fumes and buildings. The chief target organ is usually the brain, and the commonest symptoms are spaciness and difficulty concentrating. If zinc is deficient in another enzyme (alcohol dehydrogenase), the spreading phenomenon can occur. If it's deficient in other enzymes, there is abnormal gene repair, vitamin metabolism, enzyme synthesis, membrane integrity, etc.

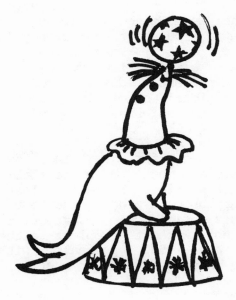

To balance one's nutrients requires:

    (1) excellent biochemical guidance

    (2) reduction in chemical load and improvement
        in diet (the two things that probably caused
        it in the first place)

    (3) periodic assessment, since nothing that is
        alive is a static phenomenon.

Now, recall zinc is only one mineral and is in over 90 enzymes. I've only given you a brief sketch of the symptoms that 5 of those enzymes could produce if someone were zinc deficient. You can clearly see that a hidden zinc deficiency can be the perfect set-up for developing chemical sensitivities, as well as the emergence of other sensitivities to pollens, dusts, molds, foods, Candida, and additional chemicals. This spreading phenomenon creates the universal reactor, sensitive to everything.

In order to check for a zinc deficiency, however, a physician must be aware that a regular serum zinc will not suffice. A special test of red blood cell or erythrocyte zinc is the test of choice that will show this deficiency. Correction of the deficiency is not without problems either. In treating well over 500 patients with zinc deficiencies, we have seen that it must be done very carefully with a great deal of appreciation for the biochemical interaction. For example, molybdenum, manganese, copper and other minerals can all displace each other from crucial enzymes. If a zinc deficiency is treated too aggressively or incorrectly without the proper balance, the patient, in a month or two, will have deficiencies of copper, molybdenum, or manganese. These in turn have their own lists of voluminous symptoms. For example, copper is in over a dozen enzymes. A copper deficiency might affect the enzyme ascorbic acid dehydrogenase, so that one cannot break down vitamin C or ascorbic acid into its first usable metabolite.

Another facet that came from this research was that in most people, very high levels of zinc were required to correct deficiencies slowly over several months. No one would dream of using, for example, levels of zinc ten times the normal RDA without having blood tests available to monitor not only the progress of the zinc, but that of the copper, manganese and other minerals that can be involved in this delicate balance.

In the beginning when a correction is begun, levels are necessarily unbalanced, since the individual is already unbalanced with his deficiency. Later on when the correction has been made, and the balance can be checked in the blood, then maintenance levels of nutrients can be prescribed, which have a far different balance than a corrective prescription. If the corrective prescription is taken beyond the prescribed time, the pendulum swings to the opposite side and imbalance results in other nutrients.

We are entering an era where doctors will need to start learning molecular biochemistry and the science of nutrition. For due to the over-work of the body's chemical detoxification system from our 20th century diets and lifestyles, many people are nutritional time bombs just waiting to go off. They're missing many nutrients and are in a poor state of balance and no one knows it. They themselves know that something is wrong, though, and that they're not playing with a full deck. But they don't know how to go about finding the solution. E.I. is a product of the 20th century and it shows us that many rules of medicine are inadequately archaic. When one is already chemically overloaded, you can't treat him by giving another chemical or drug.

Many of them (like myself) will, or have, gone on to become victims of environmental illness, with reactivity to dusts, molds, pollens, Candida, foods, and many chemicals. But by correcting their nutritional deficiencies they can strengthen their detoxification enzymes once again.

How does one know if he might be a nutritional time bomb waiting to go off? Very easily. Many already sense that they do not feel vivacious, happy and enthusiastic the majority of the time. They know that there is something wrong. That is the time to find yourself an environmentally and nutritionally oriented physician, before your time bomb goes off.

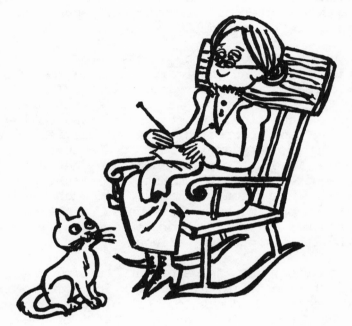

Even Granny knew a stitch in time saves nine.
It makes sense to identify nutritional deficiencies
when symptoms are nebulous and minor.

Chapter IV

DETOXICATION: THE PATH TO REJUVENATION

FOR DOCTORS ONLY. This chapter is too technical for the average reader. Most may want to skim through the technical parts and get on with their program. Later on curiosity may spur you on to return to it in more depth.

As you have seen, the body has a vast xenobiotic (foreign chemical) detoxication (also called biotransformation or detoxification) system. Starting in the liver, it extends through the lungs, gastrointestinal tract, skin, and kidneys, metabolizing and excreting foreign chemicals that enter the body everyday through contaminated air, food and water. This xenobiotic detoxication system requires a vast amount of energy and nutrients to function maximally. Although the body can heal a surprising array of wounds, diseases and broken bones, as well as broken spirits, it needs optimum health for optimum wellness.

Rejuvenation, or an apparent turning back of the hands of time definitely occurs in some people as they begin to depurate, or unload accumulated toxins that accelerate the chemistry of aging. Everyone has a particular load of toxins that is so individual that it's like a biochemical fingerprint. These toxins can be reduced, thereby reducing the stress to the body. Likewise in order to heal many conditions, an unloading is necessary.

For example, in some cases, people with E.I. cannot improve past a certain point using a good ecologic program because their cellular biochemistry or machinery has been poisoned. These poisons simply must be removed before healing can progress. These poisons can be old drugs, pesticides, medicines, or many of the thousands of chemicals we are exposed to daily in our food, air, and water. Whatever their sources, whatever their routes of contamination (absorbed through skin, lungs, or gut), once they are in the body, chemicals can act like a monkey wrench in a cogwheel, impeding normal function until they are removed. And a poorly functioning chemistry makes one more easy prey to disease and speeds up deterioration or aging.

The body has many ways of getting rid of these chemicals or detoxifying the body. (Incidentally, in science, this is more properly called detoxication or biotransformation, and foreign chemicals in the body are termed xenobiotics. At first I hesitated using such big words, but they are words you will hear in the future anyway. PCB's, dioxin and radon were unfamiliar ten years ago, but everyone has some glimmer of what they connote today. Likewise xenobiotic detoxication will roll off your lips in the future, so you might as well begin to practice.) Anyway, once a chemical has gained entry to the body, it can undergo a variety of chemical reactions in the body's attempt to get rid of it. There are many possible pathways, some good and some harmful.

Sometimes the body goofs and turns the chemical into a more dangerous or even more carcinogenic (cancer-causing) chemical. Sometimes the body has a dozen possible pathways that can be used, but chooses a particular one because the other paths are already overloaded detoxifying other chemicals that got there first. Later on it may use some of these alternate pathways and produce totally different metabolites than it did initially, and some of them are more dangerous than the initial, or parent, compound. Obviously if on one occasion you're exposed to formaldehyde, for example, and it is metabolized quickly into a harmless chemical, you'll not react. But say on another day you had

had some other exposures as well as your formaldehyde. The regular pathway might be overloaded so the formaldehyde is shunted to a different route which produces metabolites that cross into the brain and produce depression. And this is a very simplified example of the total load. Imagine what happens as you inhale and ingest scores of toxic chemicals all day and night? Sometimes a chemical is so abnormal, the body doesn't have a good chemical setup to detoxify and it stays in the body, usually as a transformed metabolite.

The organs the body uses to expel chemicals are the lungs, skin, bowel, bladder, and reproductive organs. That's it. There are no other ways to get rid of chemicals. They have to exit from one of those places.

The liver is the most active organ in transforming these chemicals so that they can be expelled. In the cells of the liver are a series of membranes called the endoplasmic reticulum (ER) where a vast amount of this chemistry goes on. This chemistry is dependent on many nutrients in order to proceed. So it seemed logical to us to look at making a nutritional detoxication program. In other words, if the nutrients which the detox pathways depend upon are beefed up enough, this should facilitate the body in detoxifying itself even against greater twentieth century environmental stresses. Such a program must be individualized to the person, however. There is no canned approach as we have available in much of medicine, because everyone is so unique.

To further complicate matters, nearly every nutrient plays a role in the detoxication process of xenobiotics. You've already seen how just one deficiency like zinc can affect every major biochemical pathway in the body, and that a deficiency of this one nutrient has far-reaching effects in terms of the body's ability or disability to detoxify. There is also a domino effect whereby its persistent lack is felt in many enzyme systems that themselves go on to further disturb other enzymes, causing many other deficiencies. Likewise, a deficiency of zinc in the xenobiotic detoxication system causes a buildup of chemicals in the liver which can further damage and stress the already ailing detoxification system. It's sort of like the branching of a tree. If one element is missing, then several other pathways are secondarily adversely effected, and then these pathways furthermore effect changes in numerous other pathways. And what is the result? The snowballing or spreading phenomenon we have so frequently seen that results in the universal reactor, or those who react to everything: molds, (which includes Candida), foods and chemicals.

One of the worse symptoms the universal reactor endures is the toxic brain syndrome. He feels exhausted, can't concentrate, spacey, dizzy, nauseated, and headachey. He feels like he's been drugged, and to complicate this nightmare, there are no blood tests or x-rays to diagnose it.

To further complicate matters, the toxic brain syndrome is not caused by just one or two things. It can be triggered by such things as an unsuspected nutritional deficiency, an emotional strain, or a heightened sensitivity to molds, food, Candida, and chemicals as well as by many other things.

We are now beginning to understand some of the biochemical mechanisms of it. Some of the most common problems are indoor and outdoor chemicals, such as the hydrocarbons. Not a day goes by where you are not exposed to these at home, at work, or in your food or water. We are beginning to

53

learn how these 20th century foreign chemicals, broadly known in the biological world as xenobiotics, can cause brain fog or toxic brain syndrome.

Common xenobiotics, or foreign chemicals, include such hydrocarbons as xylene, benzene, toluene, vinyl chloride, and trichloroethylene (TCE). These are the chemicals found in plastics, glues, paints, clothing, furnishings, food and water.

Because these hydrocarbons are lipid soluble, and the brain has a greater affinity for absorbing fat-soluble (lipid) materials than do other tissues, the brain gets higher levels of these toxins. This explains why the brain is one of the primary target organs and why baffling brain symptoms predominate. We call these cerebral symptoms, brain fog or toxic brain syndrome.

The liver, the main detoxifying organ in the body, contains certain specialized cellular components (microsomes), which participate in metabolizing foreign chemicals (xenobiotics). These cellular components process the foreign chemicals so that they can eventually be eliminated from the body. Of course these microsomes are made of membranes, so as chemicals accumulate, even the membranes that are responsible for detox get damaged. You can now appreciate the complexity of the spreading phenomenon and how difficult it is to arrest.

Xenobiotics, in the course of being metabolized, undergo several chemical changes (oxidations, reductions, degradations, and conjugations). Most of the time they are made less toxic, but occasionally they are made more toxic. Oftentimes a single chemical will have many metabolites. In other words, the xenobiotic can be broken down into a dozen different chemical compounds each with its own selective actions and side effects. (I hesitated to make some of these repetitions, but then I reminded myself that you're learning molecular biochemistry and toxicology concepts that many physicians do not know. Hence some repetition of sophisticated concepts should reinforce the learning process painlessly.)

The ability of the body to degrade (change or reduce) these chemicals depends on how many other chemicals the body is exposed to at the same time from contaminated air, food, and water. Prescription drugs and radiation also add to the burden by creating free radicals that damage membranes. It is the combination or total load and genetic factors that determine how well the body handles the additional chemicals.

The nutritional state of the individual's detoxification enzyme system and the availability of certain selected nutrients, including essential lipids, and amino acids, also affect the ability of the body to break down these foreign chemicals.

Trichloroethylene as an example

Take trichloroethylene for example. It's an all-purpose xenobiotic and, like formaldehyde, is difficult to avoid in everyday living. It's widely used in industry and is an intermediary of many chemical reactions.

It is an anesthetic, a degreaser, a dry cleaning fluid, an intermediary of plastics, oils, glues, and a common drinking water contaminant. It is one of the "inert ingredients" of pesticides, and is even used in the food industry to decaffeinate coffee and tea.

TCE, like many other xenobiotics, is broken down with the first pass through the liver into several byproducts. One of these byproducts is a chemical family called epoxides. Another metabolite is formic acid (formaldehyde), a potent toxin for most chemically sensitive individuals.

Then there are further pathways that epoxides can take. They can attach to DNA. When this happens, drastic changes may occur in our genetics which can result in mutation. It could also potentially cause the following: liver toxicity, kidney toxicity, brain toxicity, suppression of the immune system, teratogenesis (birth defects), environmental illness, accelerated aging, or even cancer.

Or other trichloroethylene byproducts can attach to glutathione and eventually be excreted in the bile. Then again, other trichloroethylene by-products can be converted to aldehydes. Aldehydes are cell toxins which start the formation of free radicals, cross-linking, and membrane destruction. These three processes have to do with the chemistry of aging, chronic degenerative diseases and cancer.

Last, but not least, trichloroethylene can be converted into chloral hydrate, a hypnotic or sedative better known as "Mickey Finn" or "knock-out drops". In the <u>Physician's Desk Reference</u> (PDR) (a book describing dosages and side effects of all prescription drugs), the list of side effects reads like any typical patient with environmental illness (E.I.) All the symptoms of brain fog are present plus peripheral neuropathy (numbness and tingling) and almost any other symptom you can think of.

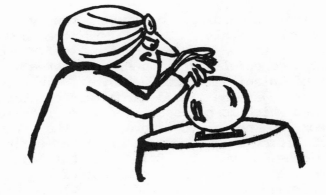

No one knows which biochemical pathway a particular chemical will take in your body on a specific day. In people whose detox systems are overloaded, common everyday chemicals often breakdown into substances toxic to the brain like chloral hydrate (the old "Mickey Finn").

Candida and Detox

Remember, alcohol, inhaled chemicals and Candida add increased aldehyde. And in the brain, it can cause the toxic brain symptoms of E.I. (spacey, dopey, exhausted, numbness and tingling, depression for no reason and more). So a drink of alcohol, for example, can put further stress on the detoxification mechanisms, and increase the acetaldehyde levels of an already compromised system and increase the Candida symptoms. That's why people with E.I. can't drink much, while everyone else is having a merry old time.

Candida, according to Truss' theory, raises acetaldehyde levels; Candida in the bowel can contribute to a malabsorption of specific nutrients, especially vitamin A, and increase levels of alanine which inhibit intracellular levels of cysteine (needed for further glutathione production which is necessary for detoxification). And so you begin to appreciate the tremendous chemical effect and why people with no training in the biochemistry of E.I. are baffled by our symptoms. But it all fits so beautifully. Look at the hundreds of people who became less chemically sensitive as soon as they treated their Candida. They merely began to reduce their total load or total body burden.

To reiterate, aldehyde production can come from many sources: trichloroethylene, alcohol, and Candida, as well as many other aldehyde precursors such as auto exhaust, formaldehyde, etc.

Therefore, as you can see, understanding the biochemistry of detoxification helps one to understand the symptoms of E.I., for they are one.

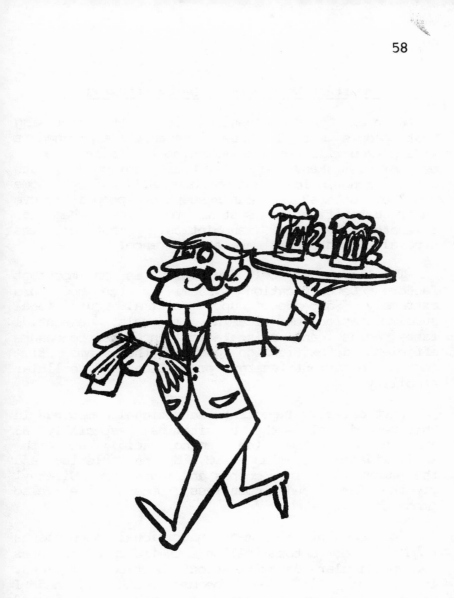

Alcohol is just another chemical that stresses the detox pathways. It breaks down to form aldehydes which can cause brain fog. Other sources of aldehydes are formaldehyde, auto exhaust, and vinylidene chloride (saran wrap, plastics). So no wonder people with E.I. can get blitzed so easily!

Important Nutrients of Detox Pathways

With all this happening, it's not surprising that people with E.I. feel like they are drugged; a wise person will begin to ask himself, is he tired or toxic. Many are really toxic; poisoned by 20th century xenobiotics. But why does E.I. affect some and not others? How can susceptible people improve their detoxification systems to allow them to tolerate levels of xenobiotics? What are the crucial elements that make a difference?

The level of cell nutrition is an important factor. Detoxification systems in the body are extremely dependent upon optimal nutritional supplementation of vitamins, minerals, essential fatty acids, and amino acids in order to ensure efficient detoxification and at the same time ensure efficient energy production and cellular stability.

Particularly important nutritional compounds in this regard include the B vitamins, especially B3 and B5, taurine (an amino acid) and the anti-oxidants, vitamins A, C, E and selenium and the minerals, zinc, copper and magnesium. Dimethyl glycine (DMG) and countless others are also important.

For some of the many nutritional supplements required for detoxification, their specific uses for particular detoxification functions follows. In places, it does become technical, and I apologize as we struggle to make complicated biochemistry understandable for everyone. Your health depends on it.

The enzyme system NADPH is very active in changing chemicals to less dangerous forms that can be excreted and is extremely dependent upon high levels of B3 (niacin). However an alarming reaction can occur if one uses it without guidance (see The E.I. Syndrome). Acetaldehyde toxicity which occurs with Candida problems and chemical overload from plastics and formaldehyde, for example, requires good levels of taurine, zinc, and B5 (pantothenic acid) to stabilize cell membranes; and aldehyde oxidase which is necessary to further metabolize acetaldehyde (a major cause of brain fog) requires molybdenum.

Since glutathione carries chemicals out of the liver and into the bile, taurine, essential fatty acids, and B5 again are needed to improve bile flow.

Mitochondrial membranes (which are the source of energy in the cell and are involved in protein synthesis and lipid metabolism) and endoplasmic reticulum membranes (structures that house the xenobiotic detoxifying microsomes) require phosphatidyl choline and phosphatidyl ethanolamine for their fluidity and function; they also need magnesium, vitamin A, beta-carotene, vitamin E, eicosapentaenoic acid (EPA), and carnitine.

Of the anti-oxidants, vitamin A stabilizes cell and organelle membranes while vitamin E grabs passing chemicals that attempt to enter the cell. Vitamin C is the only free-floating, general purpose anti-oxidant vitamin that is extra cellular (that is, it is outside of the cell protecting against xenobiotics). The rest are intracellular or inside enzymes.

Glutathione peroxidase, which helps to keep microsomal and other membrane lipids in a less toxic state, requires selenium, vitamin E, and cysteine. Glutathione reductase must have healthy levels of B2 in order to function; and liver regeneration is dependent upon vitamin B1 (as acetaldehyde and free radicals attempt to weaken and damage the liver).

Formic acid metabolism (formaldehyde) relies heavily on folic acid (a B vitamin) and aldehyde dehydrogenase (an enzyme which must have two molecules of molybdenum in it to function).

The superoxide dismutases are the body's "anti-arthritis" enzymes and protect against free radical attack that produces the aching of arthritis. They must have sufficient zinc and copper; while the mitochondrial superoxide dismutase contains manganese. And, of course, high levels of manganese must be present in order for magnesium to be absorbed, which itself is in over 300 enzymes and pathways in the body.

These are just a few of the nutritional supplements that are required for a healthy detoxification system.

It's also important to keep in mind that the detoxification system is not isolated. The way individuals see the world around them determines the way the body functions. Attitude affects the modulation of brain neuro-transmitters which in turn have an effect on the immune system, the acid/alkaline balance, the endocrine system, and the detoxication system. A healthy attitude is vital to a healthy body.

This is one reason why immunologists, internists, endocrinologists, and allergists are not able to identify and study the problems of E.I. They study isolated aspects of body physiology and rely on information that can be reproduced in test tubes. The problem is that there is no test tube that contains all the interrelated aspects of the body. The field of environmental medicine possesses no artificial boundaries and does not restrict itself to biochemistry or neurology, or immunology.

It's ironic that it's illegal to drive under the heavy influence of marijuana, alcohol, and drugs like chloral hydrate, but it's okay to drive in a new vinyl interior car behind a diesel truck. And it's alright to stop at the local dry cleaners and tank up directly on trichloroethylene. In the susceptible individual these all cause brain fog. The presence of trichloroethylene is measurable in the blood for several hours after a five minute visit to the dry cleaners. And, of course, wearing a newly dry cleaned suit keeps these levels going all day, as does working in an environment where this has been used to clean the carpets.

References in the biochemistry literature abound which support the above information, but because scientific disciplines are so fragmented, biochemists are rarely called upon to treat E.I. victims, and physicians rarely have enough time to read the journals in their own fields, much less those in nutrition, biochemistry, toxicology, and environmental medicine.

But it has been possible to detox people by improving their nutrition. Ailing chemistry can be corrected and even pushed to maximize the detox pathways.

After this, if xenobiotics persist, there are medically supervised sauna programs where chemicals can actually be sweated out. But often people returning from these programs had mineral and vitamin imbalances that had to be corrected, and they were not completely well.

But there are other methods through which the body can discharge toxins. Macrobiotics is one. Most of the persistent or stored chemicals are walled off in the fat. They must be mobilized (through exercise, sweating, weight loss, skin brushing): this turns them loose in the blood

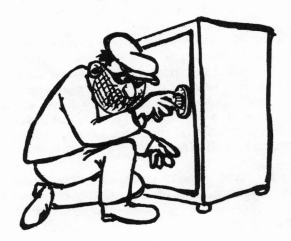

One of the secrets to getting well is to get rid
of stored chemicals or detoxicate. Macrobiotics
appears to be one such method of accomplishing this.

stream.   Here   they flow to all organs including the
liver and the brain. The result is the person may
feel very sick at this stage. It's here also that
the liver must be in tip top shape to detoxify and
excrete these chemicals to get rid of them quickly
once and for all. It's best to enter into such a
program   knowing   that   the   levels   of   crucial
detoxication nutrients are in good balance.

People   going   through   macrobiotics   will
periodically experience a cleanse   or   discharge,
where   they will have a tender liver area, for
example, and recurrence of some of their old
symptoms.   It's important at this point to try to
avoid medication to suppress the symptoms (which
adds to the chemical overload), but ride it out.
Depending in the severity of symptoms however, close
medical   monitoring   may be necessary.   One may
require blood tests at that time to be sure a
discharge   is   being   experienced, and not another
sickness. We also can do extensive analyses of the
vitamin, mineral, fatty acid, and amino acid levels
to determine the state of biochemistry and correct
it.   Also, during the course of the program periodic
checks should be made for biochemical balance to
monitor and correct any serious deficiencies
resulting from the stress on the detox system.

E.I. is a newcomer to the field of medicine and
also to the discipline of macrobiotics.   It breaks
many rules.   Ferments and grains are often not
tolerated. Often detox is delayed because foreign
chemicals, whether they be from mercury amalgams,
pesticides, or inhaled chemicals, throw a monkey
wrench in the mechanism.   And thanks to the
processed diet, many nutritional deficiencies
further paralyze the detox process. But we are
learning how to overcome much of this as we seek to
eat and live closer to nature, instead of fighting
her.

CURRENT MEDICAL THINKING IS OBSOLETE

Ecology and macrobiotics have much philosophy in common, leaving the viewpoint of "modern medicine" in the dark ages. Current disease concepts are definitely inadequate for wellness at many fundamental levels. They have served us well for years, but the time to march on has passed. The current thinking needs to adapt to the following concepts:

1. Failure is almost guaranteed with the "victim" mentality. The "Poor me, why did this have to happen to me?" leaves the person feeling powerless. Medicine further strengthens this concept of the powerless patient by having him visit a doctor-deity who has the power to prescribe chemicals with intimidating names to relieve symptoms.

    In ecology and macrobiotics, YOU are responsible for your illness, as well as your wellness. YOU are the one who ate all the wrong foods and YOU are the only one who has the power to restore YOUR wellness and to help you reach new levels of wellness. YOU have all the power. How you use it is up to YOU.

2. Every symptom has a cause. In modern medicine, drugs are prescribed to cover up symptoms. In ecology and macrobiotics, the cause of symptoms is sought. The attention is directed at how the diet and lifestyle should be altered to allow nature's healing to take place. For example, millions of dollars worth of arthritis and colitis drugs are prescribed each year. But rare is the doctor who clears arthritis by identifying that beef, potato and natural gas are the triggers. Yet these are common causes.

3. Biochemical individuality. The modern doctor needs to abandon the cookbook formula: chief

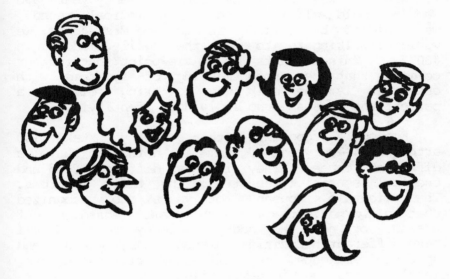

Cookbook Medicine is very popular in the western world, where all people with arthritis, for example are presumed to have the same cause, since they all have the same disease. Hence medicine is still searching for that elusive single cause.

Eastern medicine, however, now and for thousands of years and long before confirmatory biochemistry proved them correct, asserts that no two patients are alike.

complaints, history, exam, blood test, X-ray,
diagnosis, drug prescription or surgery.
Medicine sees all diabetics as one person and
all ulcers as one person. Hence, the cookbook
approach.

When I was in medical school, twenty years ago
when we would walk into a room for medical rounds,
we wouldn't be walking in to see Mrs. Jones; we
would be walking in to see the "gall bladder in
#302". This results in a viewpoint that further
commands that the gross masking of symptoms with
chemicals is the only way to bring relief to a
patient who possesses no individual identity.

Ecology recognizes that if you take 100
arthritics, every one of them is going to have a
different cause. They will have different food and
chemical sensitivities triggering their symptoms.
The orientals thousands of years ago recognized
that no two patients were the same regardless of
whether or not they had the same symptoms. We all
have different heredities, dispositions, mental and
spiritual makeups, as well as nutritional states,
intolerances, and biochemistries.

4. Masking. Medicine must think a headache is a
   codeine deficiency. Providing a serious
   treatable cause has been ruled out, we are then
   trained to merely mask, or cover up, the
   symptom, but our bodies are already capable
   of masking or adapting by themselves. That's
   the very reason most people need to do the rare
   food diet to find hidden food allergies. They
   can have arthritis for years caused by beef and
   tomatoes and not see a direct correlation until
   they unmask or unadapt by fasting five days and
   then have the food again. Then, it hits them
   like a ton of bricks because the adapting
   enzymes were fooled into thinking that they
   were no longer needed (unmasking).

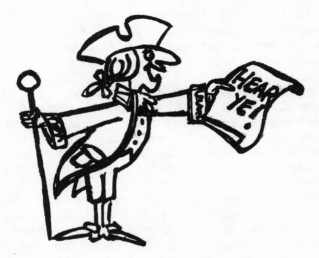

As dogmatic as medicine has become, it has been superseded by insurance companies which people have now allowed to dictate:

what illnesses they can have, how long they can have them, which doctors can treat them, and which treatments they can have.

Only people, not doctors, can change all that.

But what is the price we pay for this wonderful adaptive (masking) biochemistry so we can seemingly tolerate things that the body doesn't like? Chronic illness is the answer. The short term trade off for tolerance is long term insidious disease that builds for sometimes ten to twenty years before we know it's there. When it reaches a specific recognizable stage, then medicine steps in and diagnoses arthritis or diabetes or allergies or hypertension or cancer.

But macrobiotics can diagnose your problem long before. And what strange terms they use -- like you have hardness in your liver. What does this mean? You've eaten too many yin items like tomatoes, sugar, alcohol, medicines, and caused expansion, or swelling, of an organ that was vulnerable. It lost its elasticity and became boggy. Then you continued excesses of yang foods, as well, such as beef and salts and caused a buildup of mucus and fats so that the flow of energy was impeded, or blocked; then the organ became tight and you felt fatigued and stressed (uptight). This stagnated area became a perfect breeding ground for infection and degeneration.

Add to that the acid diet (high in meat and sugars) and synthetic vitamin D2 that is added to milk and other foods; this combination fosters calcifications that are seen in arteriosclerosis, cancers, and many other degenerative phenomena. A high acid diet draws minerals like calcium out of tissues where they belong (jawbone) and deposits them in damaged areas (vessel wall). Synthetic vitamin D2 is an unnatural product that also breaks the rules of body homeostasis or balance. In other words, it is very deleterious to the feedback mechanism so that it actually enhances calcification in weakened areas. Once we have a hardened, calcified, weakened organ, we have the seemingly impossible task before us of dissolving this hardness and restoring balance. Do you think that there is a pill in the world that can do this? But correct body pH can.

Darned if this age old method of diagnosis doesn't scoop "modern medicine" with its fancy blood tests and x-rays. Plus, this age old form of medicine fosters healing in a way that is far more effective and healthier and on a more meaningful level, as well. No doctor has the power to heal you; but YOU do.

5. <u>Total Load</u>. Medicine thinks a threshold is a level of something that all people tolerate, and that it is a stationary value; in reality, it is neither of these. That's why some physicians get crazy when we tell them we're reacting to the new carpet glue, while the rest of the office doesn't even notice it. Plus they really question our sanity when our reactions are not consistent: we react one day but not the next, or have a headache one week and nausea the following. They are totally unaware of the detoxication biochemistry, when in truth when the detoxication system is stressed to the maximum, a seemingly insignificant exposure can be intolerable and the symptoms can fluctuate daily depending upon the total load to a system at any moment.

And don't forget we also have a total mental load, as well. We all carry mental trash from years ago right up to two seconds ago that colors our reactions. Isn't it time to do some mental housekeeping as well? Start by working on forgiveness --- of yourself first, then others.

Macrobiotics recognizes both the mental and physical total load. It recommends cottons, clean air, and healthy thoughts. The reason it recommends such seeming inconsistencies like natural gas is because of the electromagnetic fields produced by electric appliances. These can interfere with the body's own electromagnetic

fields and detract from health. The problem is
with us. We have gone so far down the tubes that
we no longer tolerate gas; but people increase
their tolerances to it as they improve through
macrobiotics. At this point, because some of us
may never be truly healthy until we get out of gas
to allow healing, I cannot recommend that we use
gas. I am not inclined to ever use it again, even
though I tolerate exposures that I couldn't in the
past. I'm not sure how far we can push our
twentieth century bodies.

6. Likewise, bipolarity is unrecognized by
   medicine while it is a fundamental guiding
   principal established by environmental
   medicine. When at first bodies are
   overburdened with a foreign chemical or wrong
   food, the adaptive mechanisms come to the fore
   (masking). People feel good and many (as I
   was) are in a stimulatory phase where they are
   really hyped up with energy. As the
   detoxication and coping mechanisms become
   exhausted, end organ failure starts and they
   slip into the depressed phase, never dreaming
   that the things that made them feel so great
   could ever be the cause of such intolerable
   symptoms now. Hence, they set off on wild
   goose chases looking for everything and
   anything except the real causes that were right
   under their noses. And you can see how the
   initial stimulatory phase that made them feel
   good could be quite addicting. They
   unknowingly crave the very thing that
   eventually makes them worse. This leads to a
   downward spiral of obesity and/or other
   worsening and accumulating symptoms.

For example, Kate craves ice cream. She feels
great when she has it. Eventually she has ten
unwanted pounds, chronic tiredness and congestion.
She doesn't find this out, however until she avoids
all milk and sugar for one week and then
reintroduces it.

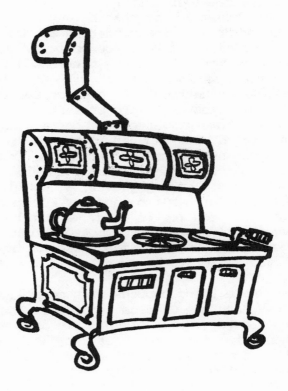

Nothing is perfect, including macrobiotics. Sure it would be wonderful if we could cook with wood or modern gas, but many of us have been so damaged by 20th century chemicals that we're intolerant of them. Avoid microwaves, as well, for they produce more of a disruption of the life force in foods than the electromagnetic fields of electricity.

7. Always remember that the pendulum swings.
   What this means is that balance is not a
   static or stagnant condition as "modern
   medicine" would have you believe. Remember
   when we were correcting nutrient deficiencies?
   At first we had to start with alarmingly high
   levels of nutrients to correct severe
   deficiencies that were present. Within a month
   or so, however, after the correction had been
   monitored, we then had to make a drastic change
   in your nutrients and switch you from a
   corrective to a maintenance level. If we had
   stayed on this high level, we would have
   created further imbalances. For example, if
   you had been low in zinc, we would have
   eventually knocked the bottom right out of your
   copper, molybdenum, manganese, or magnesium, or
   maybe all of them.

   The same thing happens with people who think
   they have the Candida syndrome. They start out
   on a sugar-free, ferment-free diet and feel
   wonderful for a month or two, but eventually
   they don't feel so hot anymore because they're
   having too much meat in proportion and have
   created a different type of imbalance. The
   same thing will happen with macrobiotics. You
   will start out on a more strict diet, but if
   you stay on this, with time you would not feel
   as well. You will need more variety and fewer
   restrictions, and you will need to balance
   your diet periodically with seasons and your
   body's demands.

   At this stage, you may be asking yourself "What
if I fail at macrobiotics?" If you've read through
all of the recommended materials, and you have

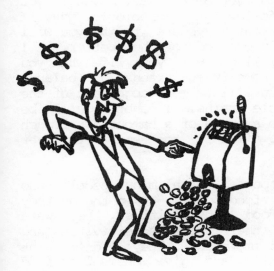

Life is a gamble, but there's no such thing as a loser if you are constantly educating yourself.

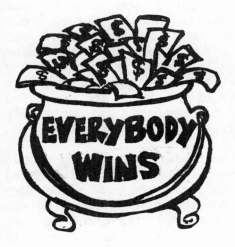

Even if macrobiotics isn't for you, you will continue to benefit after a trial, because of what you will have inevitably learned about yourself.

given it a fair shot for three to six months, I don't think you could ever be a loser. Even if you should not choose to follow the macrobiotic way, I think that through your exposure to it, you will have become irrevocably changed for the better. I don't think a week will go by in your life when you won't think of having some fresh greens to balance yourself out, and you will be more cognizant of the need of increasing whole grains. I doubt you'll be able to go back to a lunch of a hamburger, french fries and a milkshake. You're too smart to ever fall for that again.

The same thing happened with many people who looked at the rare food diet. Even though they knew they had hidden food sensitivities, they were content in ignoring their food sensitivities and being 50 or 75 percent improved. They didn't want to go that extra mile and give themselves food injections or carefully balance their diets so that they could attain further improvement. Nevertheless, they sustained a permanent marked change in the way that they ate. Once you experience a more healthful diet, you are forever changed. You find yourself holding off on wheat for a day or two if you had been overdoing and not feeling up to par. For you have learned to listen to your body, and after all a sloppy rotation is far better than none at all. As opposed to before when you were at the mercy of the food industry and their artificial flavor biochemists, you can't help but eat more thoughtfully.

Over the years, I have encountered many people that I hadn't seen for years and I anxiously asked how they were coping with their symptoms since they had left the program and what was happening in their lives. The majority of them told me that they had learned so much about foods and chemicals that they were able to handle their symptoms now without injections. Granted, they weren't at 100 percent, but they were doing so much better than they ever had before, that they were content with this level of wellness and optimistic that they could improve it with further environmental and dietary controls.

Remember, we only ever have two possibilities in medicine, and that is to medicate or educate. When I see these people, I know we were successful in educating them, because they are off all medications and they are masters of their own destinies.

Chapter V

BACKGROUND & BALANCE

ARE YOU EATING OUT ON A LIMB?

So you see that medicine customarily relabels symptoms and then finds a treatment to extinguish these symptoms. If you complain of a headache, chronic diarrhea and pain, inability to concentrate and chronic postnasal drip, you might receive such labels as migraine, irritable bowel syndrome, depression and atopic rhinitis. These are medical terms for exactly what you've already told us. Then various chemical drugs are prescribed to mask or inhibit the symptoms. The underlying causes, however, are rarely looked for and even less rarely found. If you complain too loudly about too many symptoms or symptoms that defy diagnosis, then you're warned that you're approaching hypochondriasis and may find yourself seated on the psychiatrist's couch.

Medicine, a long time ago, gave the unspoken message that you can eat, drink and breathe whatever you want; that we have a pill for everything, and you have very little control over anything. Furthermore if you are kept in the dark, this helps maintain medical mystique and dependency; hence fancy names for symptoms and drugs to maintain this distance and mystique.

But on the contrary, when the body breaks down and manifests a symptom, we should not lament and run for medications to mask the symptoms. Instead, we should rejoice, for our early warning system is beautifully operant. It tells us we are not in optimum balance and should do a good balance check to determine the cause before worse symptoms appear.

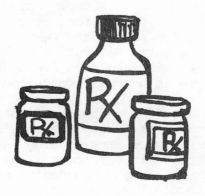

or

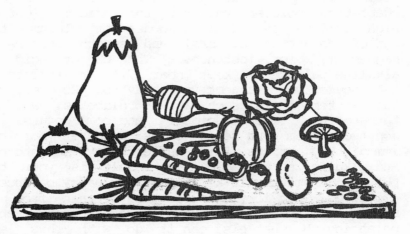

"Let your food be your medicine"

Hippocrates

Some people do not even have good early warning systems. They appear healthy for years, thoughtlessly eating whatever comes along, then suddenly they have a kidney stone or cancer. If you use all your income for vacation, you don't have any left for paying the rent. Likewise, if we eat for pure pleasure, without thought, we do not create a biochemical balance for optimal health and eventually there is a breakdown called illness.

The body has many buffer systems. These are chemical reactions that keep the body's pH, or acid and alkaline balance from going astray. If the body becomes too acid or too alkaline, coma and death result. If you suddenly down seven cola drinks, even though these are very acid, you don't die from acidosis. Why? Because your body has a marvelous chemical buffering system where it "robs Peter to pay Paul". Much like masking and adaptation, however, you pay the price. Chronic high acidity can deplete bones of calcium (it is one of the actual buffers) and smooth muscles of magnesium, for instance. The pH or acid and alkaline balance is kept near 7.43 regardless of the abuse you subject your body to. However, when the system fails such as in diabetes, a life threatening, severe acidosis and coma occurs. You don't die from your seven colas because your body immediately brings this buffering system into play and alkalinizes the acid. The result is your body pH, or chemistry is kept in a very happy balance at all times. But if you unload this strain from the body so that it doesn't have to worry about balancing pH, what else can it do with this left-over energy, but start to heal? Healing is a phenomenon that the body does naturally by itself. But it only uses biochemical energy to heal after the functions of pH balance and detoxication have been partially satisfied.

Americans in the 20th century, due to many socio-economic trends, eat on the far ends or

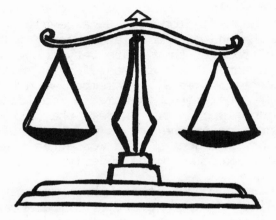

Your body is performing a constant balancing act. Salty meats (contractive) are balanced by gooey sweets (expansive), for example. Cravings result if you don't balance.

extremes of the balance scale. They eat mainly foods that are processed and contain pesticides, emulsifiers, preservatives, dyes, stabilizers and other chemicals in them. For many foods, often as much as one third of the nutrients have been removed during this processing. Also, tastes have changed in the last decades, as our modern food technology has developed. As a result, people eat way out on the end of the balance beam. They have very salty foods, they have very fatty foods, and they eat a great deal of meat. To balance all this, they eat sweets. Remember with the vitamin corrections? The more extreme a deficiency was, the more unbalanced or extreme the correction had to be. A craving is the body's way of telling you it's out of balance. The worse the craving, the worse or more extreme is the underlying imbalance.

Is it any wonder that the extremes of the American diet create extreme imbalances which manifest themselves as ferocious food cravings? Just as a severe imbalance in one nutrient necessitates a highly unbalanced correction, people eating this form of "normal" extreme American cuisine find themselves with very demanding cravings, or must have specific meals at very explicit times. When they're eating on the very ends of the balance beam or teeter totter, it's a very delicate and precise balance; the slightest upset in this balance can cause disagreeable symptoms. For example, many people know that if they don't get their coffee or their candy break or their evening high ball on time, they're irritable or headachey or extremely nervous or depressed.

Or what about those who devour a huge meal with steaks (contractive) or roasts? No matter how full they are they need to have that dessert (expansive) to balance them into a state of satiety.

However, if we bring our eating habits down nearer to the fulcrum, or the center of the teeter totter and eat a more balanced diet (one that is

closer to nature and is more replete with the
vitamins, minerals, amino acids and essential fatty
acids and don't overload the system with
unnecessarily high levels of fat, salt, sugar and
meats), a strange thing happens. Instead of the
body working maximally all the time to balance or
buffer itself, it's able to use this energy for
healing.

Since foods vary in pH, all meals produce a
resultant total stress on this buffering system.
When the stress becomes too chronic, we get
symptoms. For example, the diabetic prior to coma
may have had a tough time healing cuts, may have
gotten infected easily or had to have a root canal
or had a bladder infection. Or he was frequently
exhausted. But unfortunately nebulous symptoms can
mistakenly be confused for hypochondriasis since
they don't lend themselves to easy diagnosis. In
essence, however, they represent the best
opportunity to intervene before the condition
worsens, for they are signs that one is headed for
disaster.

So if you find yourself with a problem that
just doesn't seem to be able to be totally cleared,
it would certainly seem logical to consider
investigating macrobiotics. After all, who needs
to be eating out on a limb when the conserved
biochemical energy can be funnelled into healing?

Uncontrollable cravings, recalcitrant Candida
and chronic symptoms may all indicate that you're
eating on the edge of disaster, forcing your body
to perform an overly stressful balancing act
everyday.

Who would dream of going to the doctor for food
cravings? You'd be certain to be ridiculed or
manipulated into feeling like a hypochondriac. Yet
it's a true symptom of being "out on a limb" or too
far from the fulcrum of balance. Take someone who

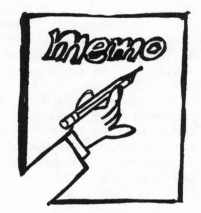

Remember, persistent Candida is not a disease. It is a symptom that your body chemistry is out of balance. Once you are healthy or balanced, you can't get Candida even if you take antibiotics, and the cravings disappear.

loves a good steak and salty cheeses. In order to buffer, neutralize or balance this very contractive food, he will crave sweets, fruits, alcohol or feel extremely edgey and depressed and resort to medications. These are all very expansive. He keeps this balance going with little margin for error, always balancing his acid and alkali, and his yin and yang.

You can tell how precarious his balance is, by how embarrassingly bizarre his carvings are, or how urgent it becomes that he get his "fixes". The urgency stems from the fact that with the slightest upset in his balancing act, he begins to decompensate and feel awful. It's analogous to the withdrawal phase of an addict, for he can feel that desperate.

This balancing act requires a lot of biochemical energy and since we never get something for nothing, there is always a price to pay. The price is lessened adaptability to the environment, premature aging, and the onset of chronic symptoms. Excess strain on the chemistry overutilizes pathways and their nutrients. This strain can come from environmental chemicals, balancing an overly acid diet and/or nutrient deficiencies from eating processed (nutrient-depleted) foods.

Take the persons who say they just can't get rid of their chronic Candida. They feel they're walking on a tightrope because they must watch their ferments and sweets very carefully. We often find they do not possess a full compliment of nutrients when we check their blood levels of vitamins and minerals. We find they are grossly deficient in some of them even though they have been on seemingly good programs. Part of the reason (aside from food processing, depleted soils, and irradiation of foods, etc.) can be from the added biochemical stress of ambient chemicals. We're the first generation ever exposed to so many chemicals. All bets are off as to how the body will respond.

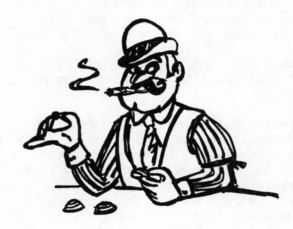

     If you're not playing with a full deck, you
will have persistent symptoms. You must have a
full complement of nutrients, balanced meals, and
have unloaded xenobiotics in order for your
biochemistry to operate smoothly.

But bear in mind there's always a reason for persistent Candida. It should never last more than a year with treatment. If it does, there is still something missing. The biochemistry is not balanced. Some of them need injections to the newer molds that we researched and published in the Annals of Allergy, (1982, 1983, and 1984) to keep their symptoms in check. More importantly, whatever the missing factor is that is required to reduce their total loads and restore balance, by not being able to totally get control of a symptom, suggests that they are pushing their buffering systems to the maximum.

The solution: do not eat so far out on a limb but closer to the fulcrum. This serves to lessen the over-worked buffering system and thereby allow the body to heal. This in turn initiates the reduction of other symptoms and lessens cravings and intolerances.

In other words, if every meal is carefully balanced to be in tune with the body, the extra energy needed for healing is suddenly available, since it is no longer needed for the chronic balancing act.

Macrobiotics provides such a diet. It is the perfect rare food or diagnostic diet (as described in our book, The E.I. Syndrome), for it eliminates frequently ingested antigens such as milk, wheat, eggs, corn, citrus, chocolate, coffee, alcohol, beef, pork, chicken, etc. It eliminates foods on the ends of the balance scale. So what is left but foods in the middle like whole grains, steamed greens, beans, root and ground vegetables, and seaweeds.
One way of eating back in the middle of the teeter totter or balance beam is through the macrobiotic approach. It attempts to keep the body in such perfect balance, so that it has energy to

not only heal but reach new states of wellness with
improved emotional stability, optimism and even
increased metaphysical awareness.

At this juncture, you have noted the use of
terms such as expansive and contractive. In
general they tend to relate to yin and yang
concepts of macrobiotics. Although neither is
precise, they serve as tools for us to better
comprehend what we are doing to ourselves with
foods so that we can decide on an appropriate
remedy. Acid and alkali do not relate to these, as
you will learn later.

Drawbacks of Macrobiotics

You might ask at this juncture if macrobiotics
is so wonderful, why haven't you heard about it
before and why isn't it more well known. The
reasons are self evident.

The major drawback to macrobiotics is that it
is different and we all resist change. It requires
a total lifestyle change and much reading and
studying. Another drawback is that it is not
readily available in grocery stores and
restaurants, and a third is that many people,
regardless of how much they try, would find the
taste of the food disagreeable. And it is not for
everyone. We've seen people who had violent asthma
attacks with every single grain. It simply does
not work for everyone, nor does anything in
medicine or life. Another drawback is that it can
cause social isolation if you are not organized and
in possession of a healthy sense of humor and self.
And, until you get well, it requires frequent
monitoring, nurturing and evaluation so that it can
adapt to your needs as you progress toward
wellness.

In the initial corrective or healing stages, it is restrictive of oils, nuts, fruits, meats and other things for some people. But this is temporary as were the corrective stages of the nutritional programs.

The advantages, however, are that we have seen many problems improve that we were powerless to help. We also found that within a few short weeks many of the cravings disappeared and many incidental symptoms melted away, such as warts that had been present for years, or morning arthritic stiffness.

We've watched it melt away severe asthma, eczema, chemical sensitivity, the toxic brain syndrome (which includes everything from depression, exhaustion, inability to concentrate, spaciness, poor self-worth, undirected anger and hostility, dizziness, mood swings and much more), as well as non-healing injuries such as chronic low back pain, shoulder injury, and hip arthritis. We've seen people intolerant of non-phenol, non-glycerine injections and intolerant of any corrective vitamins become better. They cleared in spite of not being able to take injections, became more tolerant of chemicals, and even corrected their vitamin and mineral deficiencies. The seaweeds, for example, are rich in minerals. But any natural approach like macrobiotics takes longer than a correction with store bought nutrients.

Macrobiotics doesn't make any money for drug companies, physicians, or hospitals. It takes control of health out of the physicians' hands and puts it in the hands of patients. The trained physician becomes your consultant and can direct you to macrobiotic counselors and cooking instructors to help you, and can monitor and guide your progress. But you are the one who determines whether the patient is compliant.

Also, you avoid grocery stores and restaurants by opting for chemically less contaminated whole foods. It's actually less expensive to eat the macrobiotic way and, of course, far less expensive than organic rotated diets.

The pros and cons of eating macrobiotically are as varied as your imagination. For example, if friends invite us to dinner and nervously ask my husband what I can eat, he'll casually reply, "Have you mown your lawn yet? She'll just graze for a while." Spring dandelions do provide a wealth of nutrients and can usually be found in organic form.

How long the macrobiotic way is needed is an individual decision. If one decides to stay on, there are problem areas that deserve monitoring, such as ruling out vitamin B12, zinc, fatty acid, folic acid, thiamine, and vitamin C deficiencies, or an excess of salt. We have seen abnormal levels of copper and thiamine, for example in new newcomers. Although most people improve monthly by stages, some rare individuals require a couple of years to change.

_____ _____ _____ _____ _____ _____ _____

Copy, fill out completely and bring with you the following questionnaire for your first consultation. Also copy and bring the list of food choices. But be sure you have read this entire book before your consultation.

Let's see what your current balance looks like:

DIET QUESTIONNAIRE

Name_____

Date_____

Write out your four most typical breakfasts.

1. _____   _____
   _____   _____
   _____   _____
   _____   _____

2. _____   _____
   _____   _____
   _____   _____
   _____   _____

3. _____   _____
   _____   _____
   _____   _____
   _____   _____

4. _____   _____
   _____   _____
   _____   _____
   _____   _____

Do the same for lunch.

1. _____   _____
   _____   _____
   _____   _____
   _____   _____

2. _____   _____
   _____   _____
   _____   _____
   _____   _____

3. _____   _____
   _____   _____
   _____   _____
   _____   _____

4. _____   _____
   _____   _____
   _____   _____
   _____   _____

Do the same for dinner.

1. _____   _____
   _____   _____
   _____   _____
   _____   _____

2. _____   _____
   _____   _____
   _____   _____
   _____   _____

3. _____   _____
   _____   _____
   _____   _____
   _____   _____

4. _____   _____
   _____   _____
   _____   _____
   _____   _____

And your commonest snacks or in between meal treats.

1. _____

2. _____

3. _____

4. _____

5. _____

6. _____

7. _____

8. _____

9. _____

10. _____

11. _____

12. _____

How long have you eaten this way?

What type of diet preceded this one and for how long?

Rate your meals by percentage. (The total percentage for each numbered category should add up to 100%.)

Grains (a whole grain is one that is still alive. You could sprout it in water and it would grow. Organic brown rice is a whole grain).

1. processed _____, whole* _____, organic _____

Source

2. grocery store _____, restaurant _____,
    health food store _____, garden _____

3. cooked _____, raw _____

Food choices

4. repetitious diet _____, random _____,
    rotated _____, solo foods(mono rotation) _____

Liquids consumed in a day (other than food)

5. over 6 cups _____, 3-6 cups _____,
    0-2 cups _____,

If you could feel like you want to tomorrow, list in order of preference the symptoms you would like corrected, and the number of years each has been present.

Symptom   # years you have had it

1. _____   _____

2. _____   _____

3. _____   _____

4. _____   _____

5. _____   _____

6. _____   _____

7. _____   _____

8. _____   _____

9. _____   _____

10. _____   _____

How many physicians have you consulted over the years for the sum duration of these symptoms? _____

Approximately how much money have you spent on medical bills for all of this? _____

Roughly what percent of this money was for:

        prescribed medicines   _____
        over-the-counter medicines   _____
        doctor visits   _____
        blood tests   _____
        X-rays   _____
        surgery   _____
        hospitalizations   _____
        other   _____

How much productive time was lost from work or school due to these symptoms and consultations?

How many times do you urinate in a day? _____
　　　　　　　　　　defecate? _____
　　　　　　　　　　cough? _____
　　　　　　　　　　wheeze? _____
　　　　　　　　　　sneeze? _____
　　　clear your throat of mucus? _____
　　　sniffle and snort mucus? _____
　　　# hours sleep you need _____

Do you have headaches? _____ How often?* _____
　　nasal congestion? _____ _____
　asthma/bronchitis? _____ _____
gas/bloating/indigestion?

diarrhea/constipation? _____ _____
　　　　　arthritis? _____ _____
　　　　　　fatigue? _____ _____
　　　　toxic brain? _____ _____
　　　other (state) _____ _____

* Use Code:

　　D = daily symptom
　　W = weekly symptom
　　M = symptom occurs at least once a month
　　S = sporadic, less than monthly

Do you know of any problems you have ever had with

your liver   _____
     gall bladder   _____
     pancreas   _____
     spleen   _____
     kidney   _____
     lungs   _____
     large intestine _____
     small intestine _____
     heart   _____
     circulation   _____
     glands   _____
     skin   _____
     bones   _____
     brain   _____

Comments:

Name_____ Date_____

Copy this questionnaire, fill it out and bring it
with you for your consultation with the doctor.

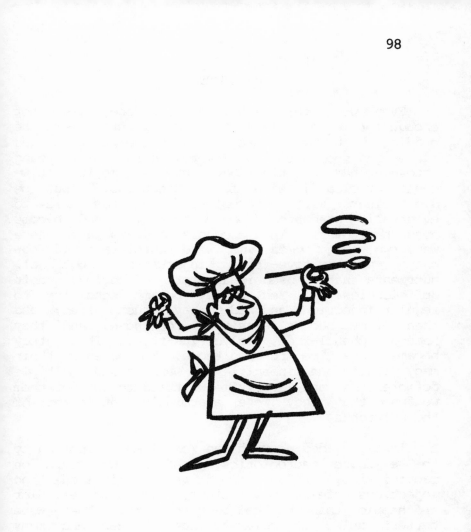

If you can't change your cooking and eating for 6 months, you're not ready to get well. You'd better explore why you need to hang on to your illness.

99

MY STORY

Even when this is all said and done, it was not
enough for me until I saw the actual proof of the
pudding with my own eyes. And the proof emerged
slowly and sporadically. Several years ago a young
attorney had colitis that surprised me in that we
could not clear it with food injections. But he
did clear with macrobiotics and was able to
eventually graduate from macrobiotics and become
even healthier. Then a couple of years later there
were two young women who were intolerant of not
only preservative-free injections, but all
nutrients that we used in attempt to correct their
deficiencies. Yes, they became sensitive to
regular injections and had to have phenol-free; and
then they become sensitive to those, and they
needed phenol-free, glycerine-free. Then they
became sensitive to even those. We looked at their
many vitamin and mineral levels and found multiple
deficiencies and everytime we tried to correct them
we found that they were alarmingly intolerant of
the nutrients.

This provided us with an excellent opportunity
to evaluate macrobiotics. After two years on
macrobiotics, these two gals required no
injections, fewer medications, and were healthier
and happier than they had been in years. They were
better able to tolerate natural gas and many
chemicals that they were intolerant of in the past,
and had indeed reached new levels of wellness. One
became pregnant, having had several miscarriages in
the past. A beautiful baby was the result. The
other was able to work in a cancer hospice, because
she was no longer restricted by her chemical
sensitivities.

Gradually, other people who were highly
chemically sensitive started evaluating the
macrobiotic process and started seeing some of
their symptoms melt away. Having had nearly every
diagnosis possible, I have always been the Guinea

pig for every new endeavor in the office; it became evident that sooner or later I would evaluate the macrobiotic process.

However, I was at a stand still at that point, because my years of symptoms were clear with ecologic management; intolerable migraines, chronic sinusitis, exhaustion and depression for no reason, chronic back pain for 15 years (after I had broken my back jumping horses), asthma and extreme chemical sensitivity leading to the toxic brain syndrome and painful muscle spasms all were clear.

I was healthier and stronger than I had been in many years that I could remember and tolerating progressively more environments and foods all the time. In fact, that year I had lectured in four countries and a dozen U.S. cities, all the while maintaining a very busy practice, writing a 650 page book, a dozen health magazine articles, and teaching in advanced courses around the country for physicians learning environmental medicine.

Then, as fate would have it, I broke a tooth on a nut shell. I was deathly afraid to have any additional mercury in that tooth, since mercury had been one of the factors that had contributed to the downfall of my immune system years before; so I elected to just ignore it.

After more than a year, my dentist insisted that I make some sort of commitment and decide on how I was going to patch up that tooth. After researching the pro's and con's, I found that all porcelain crowns and gold inlays required acrylic bonders or glues. These were deadly to me; they made me irrationally depressed and nearly suicidal; so I figured one more little piece of mercury was probably the least of my worries.

Besides I was so much healthier, I could probably take a high level of antioxidants and flush out the mercury, since we knew so much more at this point than ever before about how to biochemically detoxify ourselves.

So I let him put a mercury filling in. Three weeks later, after two hours of windsurfing, I started to develop a slight pain in my right shoulder. I didn't think much of it. The next day my shoulder was extremely painful. I sloughed it off as not being as young as I thought I was and waited for the next day when I surprisingly had even more exquisite pain. This was so severe it forced me into a sling and to take potent drugs, which I was very happy to finally have been off.

After a month of being in and out of a sling and five months of severe pain, I called a friend of mine in Chicago, who specializes in amalgam problems. When I called, I said, "Tom, I'm only going to tell you two things; one,I had an injury to my right shoulder, but the pain was way out of proportion to what I actually physically did to the shoulder, and two, it hasn't gone away in five months.

He said, "Right shoulder? I'd look at your right lower posterior molar" and I said, "You've got it!" He had known exactly what tooth I had had a mercury amalgam in because the shoulder was in the same meridian, or Chinese acupuncture line, as the tooth that had the amalgam. I didn't even tell him I had had any tooth problems or any fillings, but by knowing where these meridians go, he knew what tooth should be scrutinized as a hidden cause.

The meridians are separate from blood vessels, nerves or lymphatics. They are part of an energy and electrical system which can be manipulated via acupuncture needles to induce anesthesia for example; enough to enable a New York City reporter to have his appendix out while fully awake and sipping a cola. When poisonous metals like mercury interrupt these energy channels, disease can result in any area relating to the disturbed meridian.

At that point in time I became very nervous, because I thought I would have to have the tooth extracted or have the mercury replaced with gold and glues. And if I chose gold I would have a mouth containing mixed metals (other amalgams and the new gold) which are capable of setting up tiny currents and creating new problems. Then I remembered my macrobiotic wish that I could be a Guinea pig to work out some of the bugs of this additional approach for those who might need it.

So I swallowed my medical pride and went to a macrobiotic counselor who told me many strange things and did diagnostic things that were very foreign to me as a medically trained physician. She looked in my irises, she looked at my palms, she jumped on the floor and showed me some yoga exercises that I should do and then she began to tell me the ways that I should change my diet.

After I left her, I was highly confused, but equally determined. I went to the health store and bought all of the strange looking seaweeds, beans and grains and root vegetables that she had recommended. Fortunately, at the store they labeled the contents of the bags or I never would have even known what they were when I had returned home. Some of the things were disgusting looking; 90% of them I had no idea what they even were or how much I should buy or what to do with them. The people in the store, however, were very helpful.

At home, I called a friend who was well-versed in macrobiotics and she came over and helped me cook my first meal.

Some of the foods tasted wretched, but I ate them because of my commitment. There was a tea that was made out of fuzzy seaweed that tasted like dead fish had been rolled in it. That was to help kill my presumed intestinal parasites. There was another tea that looked like it was made out of orangey red flower petals and that was to calm me down when I got witchy and irritable (who me?). Some of the seaweeds smelled like low tide at the harbor and while I was cooking them, eating them was furthest from my mind.

I spent the next two days, (fortunately it was the weekend) reading and shopping. I couldn't believe how much I had to learn and at the same time I was constantly thinking how impossible this would have been for anyone else. Later that Sunday afternoon my friend took me to a local co-op and there I met other people who were also happy, friendly, and eager to help me. I also noticed they were very at peace with themselves, and with their approach to living. I was impressed by their willingness to give and share.

Within the first three weeks I began to like the foods and to get into a pattern so that I would be cooking up a big pot of grains or beans everyday to keep my supplies going. Several times daily I had to refer to my notes to make sure I had the right percentage of grains, greens, beans, seeds, roots, seaweeds and then all the special little teas, mushrooms and condiments. I was trying to learn some yoga exercises and skin brushing and trying to have positive and happy thoughts, while reading a voluminous amount of macrobiotic books on philosophy, theory and food preparation.

After three weeks I could raise my arm over my shoulder and swim overhand for the first time in 5 1/2 months. It felt so strange not to have that constant pain night and day. When something is with you 5 1/2 months and then is suddenly gone you feel naked, as though you've forgotten something. Also, I felt demonstratively calmer and more at peace. I didn't fly off the handle as easily and didn't have as much anger. When someone made an error, I didn't fly into a name-calling rage, insulting their ancestry. Instead I even floored myself by asking "Let me help you find where things went wrong and how we can prevent it from happening again." It was as though I had matured.

My chronic stomach problems that I had had the last couple of months totally went away and I had the most perfectly regular bowel habits I had ever had in my life, in spite of Candida programs and many food plans. I lost the morning stiffness that I had been having the last five years and there were other symptoms (like warts disappearing) that were definitely improved. These may seem insignificant but they are important indicators of the integrity of the immune system. Most of all I just felt so wonderful and happy and at peace.

Months later I went to my first dinner lecture at the local East/West Center. I sat down next to a cute elderly man and casually asked how he came to be eating macrobiotically. It turned out he was in his eighties (but looked younger and very vibrant) and had been told by a prominent local oncologist (cancer specialist) several years ago that he had only a few months to live due to spread of his deadly, malignant melanoma. He is totally clear of cancer today. His doctor considers it a miracle and does not refer other patients.

At this point in time, we're eagerly searching ways to make macrobiotics more palatable and easier to attain for other people, especially those interested in maximum wellness. But due to the tremendous individual biochemistry that abounds there is much personal tailoring that needs to be done for some to benefit from it. And macrobiotics itself is undergoing modifications in its philosophy, as its proponents realize you can't cram an Eastern philosophy down Western throats without modification and improving flexibility. As with any discipline there are the rigid, inflexible proponents, and then on the other side of the coin there are those who recognize the need for adaptation. At the same time, we must remember that macrobiotics extends far beyond just being a mere diet. It is a cosmic discipline extending to all relationships of a being. While this extensive an involvement may not be necessary for everyone, it surely will be for many. In fact for many, they thought the philosophy and lifestyle changes were more important to their wellness than the food!

Learning to eat the macrobiotic way is not as difficult an endeavor as it seems at first. At first it definitely appears utterly impossible and overwhelming. But in the first two months, not only was I strict, but I took my meals to Christmas parties, other people's homes for dinner and I even packed up all my foods and took them on a three week vacation to a Caribbean Island where I cooked and ate strictly macrobiotic. This was a particular chore since the island did not even have many "normal" foods, much less any macrobiotic foods. But as we know, adversity is just an invitation to grow. And this served to help me get organized a lot more quickly. And it shows that we are always capable of a great deal more than we had ever imagined.

Also at the same time, I cooked double because my husband and people that we would entertain did not care for macrobiotic foods (especially at the level of cooking expertise that I had), so I made regular food for them. Besides I was on a therapeutic or healing program, so I had restrictions and special foods that they wouldn't necessarily need to have, had they chosen to eat in the macrobiotic way.

It must be born in mind that when people are healing, however, they usually will need guidance. The more severe the illness, the more important is the expertise of their consultant and the monitoring of their needs to change as the pendulum swings. Once someone has healed, the range of foods becomes much wider. By then they will also have gained more wisdom in terms of listening to the body and interpreting its dietary needs.

Someone who has a severe illness, however, should not even think about going on a macrobiotic plan, unless he could commit himself to having no meats, wheat, sugars, processed foods, and oils for six to twelve months. Macrobiotics is a slow way to health, and as with anything that is worthwhile, it takes longer. It often takes a year or more for people to heal, depending upon the severity of their illnesses.

MACRO & DETOX

There are many phenomena about macrobiotics that have fascinated me. One area that I have been very interested in in the last few years is that of detoxification. As you know many of the people that we see with environmental illness have severe health problems because they have years of antibiotics, prescribed medications, illegal drugs, pesticides and chemicals that they have worked with stored in their body tissues.

These stored chemicals have damaged the biochemistry somehow so that environmental illness became manifest. Some people have fasted, others have done colonic therapies, others have gone to detoxification programs where they sweat intensely in saunas for several weeks at a time under medical supervision to get rid of these drugs and chemicals. All have had to do extensive environmental controls (as described in The E.I. Syndrome).

It turns out that macrobiotics is also a way to detoxify and as I see it, it seems that it's a more beneficial and safer way to do it. We have seen people with the other methods develop severe nutritional deficiencies that required careful correction. But on the contrary many people on macrobiotics have not developed nutritional deficiencies and we have watched them improve prior nutritional deficiencies without any vitamins or minerals. My vitamin and mineral levels after four months of macrobiotics were better than they had even been in the preceding years when I sometimes had to be on a couple hundred dollars worth of supplements a month. One reason is that the seaweeds are very rich in minerals. And some of these minerals are also good at displacing heavy metals like mercury and aluminum.

The detoxification stages or discharges or healing crises as they are called by people working in macrobiotics are an interesting phenomenon. What the macrobiotic people tell us is happening is that old diseased tissues are breaking down and old drugs, chemicals, mucous and bad accumulations are being expelled by the body. Therefore, severe symptoms will occur as these things come from the tissues into the bloodstream on their way out through the lungs, gastrointestinal tract, urine or skin.

These crises happen periodically until wellness is obtained. For example, a person may have his first discharge or healing crisis in about three months with severe aching and recurrence of old symptoms like asthma. He probably will have mucous in the bowel or from the nose or chest and after several days or a week or more of symptoms he will clear and feel as though he has reached a new level of wellness.

In a few more months another discharge may occur and so on. During these times the consultant is particularly useful in being able to advise them of what steps should be taken to minimize the symptoms and maximize the process. Sometimes the process may be too much for the person at that point in time and they can turn it off and wait for a better opportunity. People have detoxed preservatives from old injection sites, old drugs (the odor will appear on their skin or breath, or they will create an oil slick in the bathtub or on clothes). My sister had an ovarian cyst. She elected macrobiotics instead of surgery. In a few days the area under her compresses turned black. The cyst was declared gone by the gynecologist. A surgeon friend of mine recalls a man with end-stage malignant melanoma. It is a deadly type of cancer and had viciously spread to his liver. There was no way he could live more than 3 months regardless of what was done. He accidentally met him four years later and was astounded. The man told him that since he had been given such a grim prognosis, he decided to go macro. In a few months he urinated black for a few days and after that the tumors and metastases disappeared.

Recommended Reading

If you're contemplating the macrobiotic approach, you should start with several basic books, including the two personal accounts mentioned previously.

A Natural Approach: Allergies by Michio Kushi, plus the companion cookbook by Aveline Kushi, Cooking for Health: Allergies would make a good start for many. After a month or so then you would want to expand by selecting one of the following cookbooks and one of the books on philosophy.

Changing Seasons, by Aveline Kushi and Wendy Esko, is a basic cookbook. Others include Macrobiotic Cooking for Everyone, by Edward and Wendy Esko and Aveline Kushi's Introduction to Macrobiotic Cooking by Wendy Esko. Then you would need some fundamental books on macrobiotics, such as Basic Macrobiotics, by Herman Aihara, and The Macrobiotic Way (Michio Kushi).

If you want an inexpensive booklet that summarizes a great deal, read Michio and Aveline Kushi's Macrobiotic Dietary Recommendations. As you get more advanced and curious, you'll be driven to Macrobiotic Home Remedies (Michio Kushi), The Book of Macrobiotics (Michio Kushi), Healing Ourselves (Naboru Muramuto), Macrobiotics and Human Behavior (William Tara), Food and Healing (Anne Marie Colbin) and more.

Ms. Colbin has an excellent cookbook, The Book of Whole Meals, which will enable you to make delicious, gourmet meals for the rest of the family, some of which will not be recognized as macrobiotic. Just remember, much of what is allowed there is temporarily off limits to you.

Her two books also make a great start for someone who needs a more gradual transition into macrobiotics.

You can order most of these from the Seven Rays Bookstore, Westcott Street, Syracuse or Drumlins Pharmacy, Nottingham Road, Syracuse. But beware: many of these diet plans are for general maintenance macrobiotics, not corrective or specifically designed healing programs that will be mapped out for you after a consultation where it is determined what you will need. A maintenance program is for people who are no longer trying to heal any problems and can broaden their repertoires.

These books will give you a good foundation before your consultation on how you should be eating. There are no short cuts to macrobiotics , but fortunately for those in the Syracuse area there is an East/West Center which provides cooking classes, seminars, and a social milieu. One can purchase meals to take out and one can also go to dinner there. This organization provides a wealth of contacts to help you with your macrobiotic approach. As well, there are magazines, Macromuse and the East West Journal, which give many resources, such as books on macrobiotics and contacts in other cities.

Wouldn't it be nice if this approach became so commonplace that you could get a macrobiotic meal in a restaurant or on any airline? Indeed there already are some Howard Johnson restaurants in the country that have macrobiotic breakfasts. When I lectured in Dallas at an international symposium, I called the local macrobiotic center and had great meals sent to my hotel. And it cost far less than the plastic fare at the hotel.

As people become more aware of the fact that their health lies totally within their power, I think the macrobiotic approach, as seemingly impossible as it might appear initially, will gain in popularity. It can only do so as more people become hooked on their own wellness and start requiring their favorite restaurants to serve organic brown rice if they still want their business.

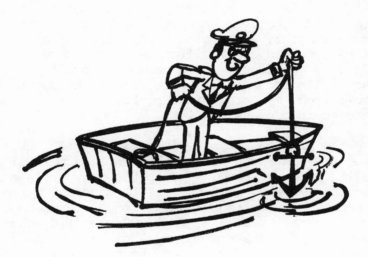

Let's weigh anchor and find out how some others have responded to the diet.

CHAPTER VI

CASE HISTORIES

P.J.'s PERSPECTIVE ON HEALING ALLERGIES THROUGH MACROBIOTICS

I experienced relatively good health as a child, and received honors for perfect attendance in my elementary and junior high school years. My family consumed meals from the four basic food groups. I especially loved cheese, fruit and ice cream. I became ill more frequently during high school, and my breathing problems were labelled "exercise-induced asthma".

While playing lacrosse in college, I developed tendonitis in both knees. The intense pain limited standing and walking. Despite many trials of anti-inflammatory medications, physical therapy treatments and cortisone injections, total healing took several years. In 1979, a bad case of mononucleosis interrupted my college studies for almost a year. I continued to have swollen glands and overwhelming fatigue, and was even more susceptible to illness.

In 1982, I happily acquired my first apartment in Syracuse, N.Y. and worked in the physical therapy department of a large nursing home. My health got dramatically worse, so I went for allergy testing and injections. I read several books and followed their advice to remove my feather pillow, stop using scented products, and eliminate some foods from my diet. Previously, my typical daily menu might have consisted of skim milk on cereal and orange juice for breakfast; mozzarella cheese on whole wheat crackers, peanuts, fruit and carrot sticks for lunch; tomato and meat sauce on noodles or white rice with a salad and Thousand Island dressing for dinner. I consumed small quantities of alcohol and pop, but had never smoked or drunk coffee. Gradually, as testing revealed allergic sensitivities, most of these foods were removed from my diet. Milk and beef were exceptions--they never seemed to cause any reactions.

My sinuses were always congested and infected. I sneezed frequently, and my sense of smell and taste had diminished. Polyps blocked my sinus cavities, inhibiting breathing, and had to be extracted several times. Each time, I vowed to do anything possible to avoid that horribly painful office surgery. I hated to rely on medications, but could not breathe through my nose without taking antihistamines and decongestants daily. I awoke 4-5 times a night to go to the bathroom and to get a drink of water for my parched mouth and throat. It's no wonder that I always felt sluggish and tired in the morning! Despite these health problems, I enjoyed my job, had a fun social life and traveled often on weekends.

My future husband, Luke, had also experienced distressing allergy problems. He had suffered many earaches and infections during early childhood. Although his condition improved temporarily after a tonsillectomy when he was six, he became ill more frequently as he got older. Working on his family's dairy farm, he consumed lots of fresh milk, hearty meals of meat and potatoes, and delicious desserts. After college and a traumatic car accident, he returned to the farm as co-manager. Non-stop sneezing attacks while working in the barn left him exhausted--it seemed that he was allergic to the cows! He also experience wheezing, incapacitating headaches and searing chest pains. Allergy injections and medications controlled the symptoms somewhat, but he continued to endure frequent colds, sinus infections, asthma, bronchitis and pneumonia. Desperate to feel better, Luke was forced to give up his chosen vocation and leave the farm. When he returned to college, some of the symptoms were alleviated. He continued to receive allergy injections for awhile, but often had bad reactions to them. Extensive tests could not detect the reasons behind his persistent headaches and chest pains.

For over a year after we were married, I took the pill for contraception. I didn't know at the time that it, like antibiotics, could upset the balance of bacteria in my system and contribute to yeast infections. I was being awakened every night by severe wheezing. Gasping for breath, I would sit up for about an hour until it subsided. This distress lasted a couple years. I was getting harder for me to work with my patients. The scents of their perfume, aftershave, powder, and cigarettes provoked sneezing and sinus headaches. I had to interrupt therapy sessions repeatedly to blow my nose.

I was referred to a conventional allergist for more testing. Desensitizing injections reduced the usual flare-up of symptoms during the spring pollen season, but overall, my condition had deteriorated. From experimenting with my diet, I knew that sugar and other refined foods caused many acute reactions. When I tried to convince this doctor that I felt that food sensitivities, especially sugar, caused my symptoms, he retorted, "You can't possibly be allergic to sugar--everyone eats it every day..." Surprised at his ignorance, I realized that I knew more about food allergies than this medical "expert"! What a waste of precious time and money...

The books I had been reading confirmed that sugar, cheese and processed foods caused many health problems. By now, I could not smell or taste at all and was rapidly losing weight. Although I was accused of being anorexic, I was eating huge quantities of yogurt, fruit, fish, poultry, lean meats, potatoes, avocados and frozen vegetables. I still had strong cravings for sweets, pizza and other foods which I had eliminated from my diet. I felt deprived at most social events and celebrations where food and alcohol were emphasized.

Gradually, I realized that the air in churches, shopping malls, new buildings and my workplace provoked nasal congestion, sneezing, wheezing, dizziness, inability to think clearly and sinus headaches. The fumes from our natural gas stove and heat, Christmas trees, and exhaust from vehicles were also implicated. We moved to an all-electric apartment and I stopped going to church and stores. It was hard to explain this to others, but Luke totally believed and empathized. He had been experiencing more headaches while working in a new office building, and was also bothered by scents and chemical fumes. In addition to sleeping at least ten hours at night, I took naps during my lunch hour and after work, but the fatigue persisted. Exasperated, I left my job to attend college part-time. I really felt alienated and cheated by my limitations.

In 1984, I went to see Dr. Sherry Rogers. At last, someone besides Luke believed that I actually experienced these symptoms. Better yet, she had confidence that she could treat me and reduce my use of medications. I underwent testing that revealed sensitivities to almost every pollen, dust, mold, hormone, chemical and food imaginable.

This syndrome of severe allergies was called "Environmental Illness" and I was classified a "universal reactor". Injections for pollens, dusts and molds eliminated the seasonal "hay fever". When hormones were neutralized, symptoms of PMS and endometriosis disappeared. Other improvements were noted when I switched from chlorinated tap water to bottled spring water. Unfortunately, I still reacted in various ways to almost everything I ate. Testing revealed that I was sensitive to almost seventy-five foods. Broccoli and rice were among the worst offenders. Daily food injections significantly raised my tolerance.

Luke accepted a new job which led us to Michigan. Once there, I discovered another enlightened medical practitioner, a dentist who was knowledgeable about the toxic effects of mercury on the immune system. He replaced all of my amalgams (silver fillings containing mercury) with plastic composites. My energy level and tolerance to foods improved immediately, and the nightly wheezing was less intense. Foolishly, I resumed eating some of the foods I had eliminated, and the recovery did not last very long.

All Winter, Luke suffered bronchitis and sinus infections, and developed headaches daily at work. Relocations to a basement office and a brand-new building exacerbated his problems. After joking about our explanations of what triggered our symptoms, the physicians could offer no solutions, only more medications.

In May 1986, my bout of pneumonia was followed by a week of immobilizing headaches. My balance and vision were distorted, one side of my face was numb, and high doses of narcotic painkillers couldn't subdue the torture. After one emergency room visit failed to detect the problem, I was admitted to another hospital. It was the worst night of my life. No tests were performed, no more painkillers were given, and I was not allowed to eat or drink anything. Unable to sleep, I begged every hour for something to relieve the mind-splitting pain. It was finally explained that the doctor feared that I had an aneurysm in my brain. Any medication would mask the symptoms and inhibit the diagnostic process. Intuitively, I knew that the problem was in my sinuses.

The next afternoon, CT scan results indicated "severely abnormal" conditions. I remained in the hospital for a week on I.V. antibiotics to treat the massive sinus infection. Further testing revealed that polyp growths densely packed all of my sinuses. Extensive surgery was required to remove the polyps, and my deviated septum was corrected. My nose hurt for months!

It had been an expensive and painful ordeal, but excision of the polyps restored my sense of smell and taste! At first, I splurged on a few treats (pizza and ice cream), but mainly favored large quantities of fresh fruit. We continued to eat lots of fish, lean beef, poultry, dairy foods, potatoes, granola and frozen vegetables. We often cooked in the microwave.

My general health deteriorated rapidly when I went to work in a new physical therapy office. My nose and sinuses became congested and my throat was so sore that I could barely talk by the end of the day. The thrill of smelling and tasting had only lasted two months. Within three months, I was back to the point where I could chew raw garlic cloves and not taste them at all. Poor health forced me to leave another job that I loved.

Luke drove me 8 1/2 hours to see Dr. Rogers.
The exhaust fumes along the highway caused extreme
lethargy and I had to use portable oxygen when we
drove through highly polluted areas, such as
Buffalo. I had recently discontinued my allergy
injections because they made my arms sore. Testing
determined that I was now sensitive to the
preservatives. Fortunately, Dr. Rogers was one of
the few physicians in the country who had
preservative-free extracts. I had everything
retested. It was expensive, but the new pollen,
dust, mold, yeast and food injections helped to
reduce the total load on my system.

The following winter back in Michigan was
frustrating for both of us. As usual, we were
exasperated that illness was controlling our lives.
When twelve different medications were powerless in
fighting my bronchitis, I was forced to re-enter
the hospital for more I.V. antibiotics and
respiratory therapy treatments. The constant, deep
wheezing returned a week later. Desperate for an
answer, I returned to Dr. Rogers. She suspected a
yeast infection in my lungs and put me on a
systemic anti-fungal medicine. Despite the fact
that I had been taking two to three grams of pure
vitamin C daily, blood tests indicated deficiency.
More supplements were prescribed.

Soon, the wheezing disappeared and I noticed a
reduction in various sinus and digestive troubles.
I tried repeatedly to eliminate or decrease the
anti-fungal medication, but the horrible symptoms
returned immediately. Frequent blood tests were
required to make sure that my liver did not sustain
any damage from the drug. I prayed that the tests
would remain normal!

Meanwhile after steadily going downhill
himself, Luke finally consented to allergy testing.

He also required the preservative-free extracts.
Fortunately, they helped his headaches and sinus
congestion almost immediately, but many other
symptoms remained.

It was absolutely ridiculous! We had quit
jobs, switched workplaces and apartments,
eliminated alcohol and many foods, done
environmental controls, endured extensive testing
and injections, replaced amalgams, drunk only
spring water, read many books, taken medication and
supplements, and spent thousands of dollars, but
still had not found the key to good health.

Dr. Rogers was the only physician who had ever
encouraged us to constantly re-assess and reeducate
ourselves about our medical problems. She had
recommended numerous books over the past four
years, but it was her suggestion to read Recalled
by Life (by Dr. Anthony Sattilaro) that changed
our lives! Inspired by this miraculous story of
healing through macrobiotics, I reasoned that if
this way of eating could dissolve his tumors, then
possibly it would have an effect on my recurrent
sinus polyps. I obtained Cooking For Health:
Allergies, by Aveline Kushi. This book was
invaluable in getting me started.

We had our first macrobiotic meal on November
11, 1987 -- Miso soup with carrots, daikon and sea
vegetables, millet, and steamed Chinese cabbage.
Luke stated that he would eat my new foods, but he
didn't want to eliminate his favorite foods from
his diet. Less than a week later, after observing
my new enthusiasm for eating, he read Recalled by
Life. It convinced him to wholeheartedly join
"the experiment". I wasn't surprised. Generally
open-minded, he was receptive to anything based on
common sense, even if it wasn't "normal" according
to others' standards.

After the first week, I realized that I no longer felt sluggish after eating supper. We went to see a macrobiotic counselor. By merely looking at my face, he could tell that I had previously eaten many dairy products. In disbelief, we listened to his claim that by changing our eating habits we could heal our bodies and totally eliminate our allergies. It seemed impossible -- until now we had only heard of ways to CONTROL allergic symptoms!

We felt hopeful as we outlined our long and short term goals. I had grown accustomed to the annoyances of frequently blowing my nose and not being able to smell and taste, but never having enough energy to do what I wanted was an endless frustration. My goals included being able to awake feeling refreshed after a reasonable amount of sleep, to have increased stamina and endurance, and a reduction in the amount of medicine and vitamins I was taking. In addition, I wanted to avoid having polyp surgery ever again.

We put our microwave in the storage closet, stopped frequenting the supermarket, and joined the local food co-op. We concentrated on chewing each mouthful of food thoroughly and stopped snacking within three hours of going to sleep. I read more, trying to figure out what the unusual words meant and how to prepare the new foods. It was astonishing -- so many nutritious foods that we had never heard of! Surprisingly, I only reacted negatively to two of the staple foods: organic brown rice and azuki beans. They provoked sinus congestion, headaches, dizziness and depression. I cooked them for Luke and substituted other grains and beans for myself.

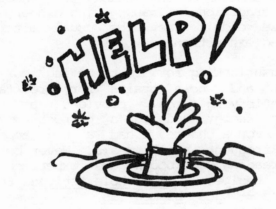

When a sound ecologic program is not enough, it makes sense to commit yourself to a trial of macrobiotics. But if Sattilaro's and Nussbaum's books don't convince you, nothing will.

By Thanksgiving, I had naturally pink cheeks for the first time in years! I learned later that this was an indication that my lungs were functioning better. Another positive sign was that in only three weeks I had cut the dosage of my asthma medications in half. It was remarkable.

Although they thought our new beliefs in foods were unusual, my family was thrilled about my improved appearance and our optimistic attitudes. With the exception of the squash, we chose not to eat the traditional Thanksgiving dinner, and for a change, we didn't feel the usual after dinner overstuffed exhaustion!

We began looking forward to having our leftover Miso soup and whole grains for breakfast. This warm, satisfying meal provides a wonderful sustaining energy and is a perfect way to start each day. For a change, I had a big appetite and consumed frequent small meals. Never before had I enjoyed reading cookbooks and experimenting with different recipes. My whole attitude toward food had changed -- once blamed as the cause of many allergic reactions, it was now viewed as the most crucial factor in my healing process.

One month after starting our experiment, we were convinced that this was the answer we had been searching for. We both felt more alert and energetic, we had clearer sinuses, fewer mood swings, more regular digestion and elimination, less flatulence, and better facial color. We had cut down considerably on vitamins and supplements, and I only required 1/4 of the usual medications to control the symptoms of my asthma and multi-focal yeast infection.

We were even more convinced of the worth of our new food choices when we survived the Christmas holidays without suffering from flus, colds and infections that plagued almost everyone around us. It was becoming apparent that our tolerance had greatly improved! We could now experience stress, exhaustion, and environmental toxins without succumbing to the illness that usually resulted.

For the first couple months, we often felt hungry and unsatisfied soon after our meals. Our digestion proceeded faster since we weren't consuming the excess fat present in the Standard American Diet (S.A.D. --- appropriately named). Gradually, our systems adapted to the switch from digesting mainly animal-quality foods to vegetable-quality foods. I no longer needed to eat constantly to feel satisfied, and we had lost our desire for meats and sweets. We had discovered some foods that we could eat in the car so traveling became easier.

After two months, I discovered that the breast cyst which had been unchanged for six years was getting smaller! I was amazed, but our macrobiotic counselor and Dr. Rogers were not -- it was said that the cyst was a result of my previous dairy food consumption and would eventually disappear. The numerous moles on my face and body also indicated the storage of excess mucus from animal protein consumption. (It is a relief to not have to worry as much about them developing further.) Blood tests revealed no more vitamins deficiencies -- my first normal results in four years!

By now, I could eat pressure-cooked, short-grain organic brown rice on a daily basis. I was delighted, since it had always given Luke a boost of energy. (He took it for lunch to work, with cooked vegetables or soup in a wide-mouth thermos.) Soon, I realized that I was able to accomplish more each day without getting tired, and I no longer needed frequent naps. In addition, I had noticed brief moments when I could smell.

I've experienced minor "symptoms of adjustment"--muscle and joint soreness--but no acute detoxification process. Luke discharged some excess mucus and toxins when he had cold-like symptoms for two weeks, (without the usual fatigue and achiness often associated with a cold). In comparison with last year, our health this winter has improved dramatically. He missed an average of four sick days per month from work then, but has not missed a single day since our dietary changes!

After marvelling at the way our lives have changed, Luke remarked, "Why did God give us the curiosity to seek the knowledge to improve our health? Maybe it's because we were meant to also guide others in their search for better health." I often shed tears of joy and amazement while reading Recovery: From Cancer to Health Through Macrobiotics, by Elaine Nussbaum. I knew that every word of her inspiring story was true, because I had felt the power of this miraculous healing myself.

But how could we get others to believe that the food was responsible? Lend them the books! Having more information has helped our family and friends to better understand our reasons for following macrobiotics, and it has motivated some of them to institute some changes in the way they eat. (It is hard to resist the thought of feeling better, looking younger, and living longer!) After following some of the principles for two months, my mom discovered an unexpected benefit--the psoriasis that had covered her knees and elbows for thirty years had almost completely disappeared. In addition, substituting various whole grains and beans for poultry, meat, cheese, and pasta made it easier for her to lose weight quickly.

Now, four and a half months since our first macrobiotic meal, this way of eating seems "normal", and we can't imagine returning to the Standard American Diet. We no longer need the expensive medications, nasal sprays, vitamins or supplements. My endurance has improved considerably. Being tired at the end of a long day no longer means that I will be exhausted and sick the next day. At least, I feel refreshed when I awaken and don't have to be dragged out of bed. (I only feel groggy in the morning if I've eaten within several hours of my bedtime or splurged on excess fruit and snack foods.) We sleep soundly and require less sleep than before. Our sinuses are much clearer—it is wonderful to be able to breathe freely again. The postnasal drip that aggravated Luke constantly for twelve years is gone, and lately I have been able to smell briefly everyday. I expect to be able to taste food eventually, and feel assured that I'll never again have to undergo that horrendous polyp surgery! We are confident that my cyst and the dark circles under our eyes will totally disappear. We have increased the number of days between our allergy injections, and anticipate the day when we won't need them at all. We have enough energy to exercise almost daily, and I find that I can do more vigorous exercise in one day than I used to be able to do in a week.

I am much less chemically sensitive, and can better tolerate being in libraries, homes with gas heat, and some stores without the fear of having an acute reaction or "spacing-out". My talents and goals were inhibited by my health limitations for many years, but I am now looking forward to fulfilling my dreams of being successful in my custom wall stencilling business.

The exhilarating freedom of improved health has created other major changes in our outlook on life. We can consider having children (without the fear that they would be severely allergic or that we would be too sick to care for them). We can save money to buy a house now that the burden of excessive medical bills is gone. I feel a sense of reverence for the food, and gratitude to all who have helped to make our recovery possible. I know that we were meant to be sick during the beginning of our adult lives, so that we might learn how to be well for the rest of our lives.

Some people remain skeptical of our new way of eating. This is not surprising, since we had tried so many remedies in the past. Besides, the choice to heal oneself without conventional medical treatment is not well supported by our society or culture. It has become accepted for people to take medication daily to temporarily relieve their symptoms, and for children with chronic infections to end up on rounds of antibiotics or have to endure ear tubes or tonsillectomies. The probable underlying cause of the problems -- what they are eating -- is usually unknown or ignored, and new problems inevitably appear. For awhile, I thought I could eat anything as long as I took my medications. It was easier to do that than investigate and change the underlying causes. However, it was my experience that the symptoms only got worse as the denial continued. I am awed that something as simple as food could be the answer to many of the complex health problems that have perplexed conventional medical practitioners for years.

Most of us are afraid of the unknown and are threatened by new ideas. It is easier to make excuses than to make changes! Being committed to wellness means letting go of stubborn ideas, beliefs and excuses. It means opening up one's mind to new ideas, and accepting the responsibility for one's own illness and recovery. There is a valuable lesson to be learned: We each have the capacity to affect our own health and destiny. What you do with that power is up to you...

P.J. Tetreault
March, 1988

A note from P.J.'s doctor: P.J. is, as you can see, a multi-talented and resourceful survivor. She points out many essential ingredients to success: (1) a willingness to persist until the key to wellness is found,
(2) optimism,
(3) love and respect of self and others,
(4) a realization that in the quest for wellness, the degree of difficulty in the solution may be in direct proportion to how much you hurt, and
(5) that food should be thought of as a friend and healer, not as the enemy we have perceived it to be in allergy.

An important warning is that many of us were not able to reduce or eliminate our allergy injections for months or years. All cases are individual. If you are not absolutely certain that you will remain on a macrobiotic program, it would be less costly and easier to extend the interval between injections to every 2-4 weeks for a year or two. Then in the event that you decide to discontinue macrobiotics, and/or that you still need your injections, you can merely tighten up the interval between them rather than completely retest.

Some people were told by macrobiotic counselors who underestimated the severity of their illnesses to discontinue their injections and they sustained life-threatening reactions because they were not ready.

— — — — — — — —

REGISTERED NURSE, REPORTING

When I was an infant in the early 1940's, it was believed that newborns had an enlarged thymus gland and many of us were given radiation treatments to shrink our so called "enlarged gland". This was done to me. Consequently , the treatment took a toll on the proper development of my immune system.

Beginning in infancy, symptoms indicated I was allergic to dairy and wheat. I progressively added to these intolerances with new allergies. Some symptoms changed through the years, but I continued to deteriorate not realizing what was happening. Now I understand that repeated exposure to antigens (foreign substances) eventually depletes key components of a person's immune system. Aluminum accumulated in my body from cooking with aluminum pots, from deodorant, baking powder, and other products containing it. Nickle accumulated in me from excessive use of margarine, and copper from an unknown source.

Throughout my life, mornings were particularly difficult. I awoke tired, feeling like I had shoveled coal all night, and lived for nap periods. Following naps, I yearned for sleep that night only to awaken the next morning as tired as I had been the previous day. This incredible fatigue was discussed with several doctors. I was told that I was fortunate to have my allergy symptoms manifested in fatigue rather than something worse such as asthma. "Which would you rather have to cope with, fatigue or asthma"? I left them feeling fortunate to have the fatigue.

My doctors recommended on numerous occasions I have surgery on my sinuses, even with this operation's low percentage of hope for reduction in infections. Fortunately I refused.

I returned from every visit to my parents home with an incredible headache and joint pains. Arthritic tests would show a 4 plus positive for rheumatoid arthritis, but none of the anti-arthritic drugs relieved the pain. I later learned my mother sprayed her home daily with Lysol. In so doing, I was exposed to phenol. This spray, coupled with the exhaust fumes on the expressway added to the high degree of toxins affecting me.

Our dog infested our home with fleas. Three weeks following the pesticiding of our home I developed low grade fevers off and on throughout each day. At this point, I concluded I needed an allergist to help me. The doctor, Sherry Rogers, told me I was "environmentally ill" with severe allergies to inhalants, foods and chemicals. I was even allergic to the chlorine in tap water. With the aid of environmetal controls, allergy shots and chemical filters (in my bedroom, office, and car), and thanks to my allergist I recovered a small percentage of health. I understood the only hope I had was to learn to control my environment in hopes of not becoming sicker than I was.

However, following one extended automobile trip with its exposures to the diesel fumes of expressways, I regressed and reacted to everything including allergy injections. The injections caused giant hives. It was a new symptom for me. This exasperating experience led me to seek alternative treatments.

One alternative I discovered was the Macrobiotic Diet. A nurse I knew, who also had been severely chemically sensitive, recommended it to me. This was a turning point. My health has been steadily improving since.

I visited a macrobiotic counselor who works with chemically sensitive individuals. She was my first experience with a holistic health approach. Using the art of visual diagnosis, like a Sherlock Holmes observation, she pinpointed many of my health problems. She observed that my kidneys were affected, based on dark coloration under my eyes, among other observations. Gall bladder and liver problems, hormones out of balance, intestines, etc. gave other indications of problems to the knowledgeable observer.

She gave me a written, "healing" diet to follow specifically designed for my condition. Seaweeds were included to help push heavy metals out of my body. Ferments and molds like mushrooms, wine, fruits, yeast containing foods, vinegar, etc. were excluded from my diet to decrease Candida. She recommended I rotate my foods as much as possible so as not to build intolerance to the new foods in my diet. Root vegetables were added to help balance the acid and alkaline content of my system. Beans and fish added protein. I started to take macrobiotic cooking classes to learn not only to cook the whole grains, beans, seaweeds, etc., but also to learn to appreciate what each food's benefits would be in helping heal.

A chronically ill person must adhere to a rigid diet to enable the body to rid itself of toxins and become better balanced. This healing can take a good deal of time depending on the severity of the condition.

Initially, when I began the diet, I experienced a "honeymoon period" when many chronic symptoms disappeared. Fatigue, constipation, irritability and depression, to name a few, left for a time.

But fatigue returns if I ingest a food substance I'm still sensitive to. Within 20 minutes of having wheat I'm sound asleep for 2 to 4 hours and exhausted for the following 24 hours. However, and increased use of whole grains that I'm not sensitive to, has given me an energy level I never dreamed obtainable. Much to my delight, I find there are no dips and peaks in my energy during the day.

The diet completely eliminated chronic constipation of 30 years' duration. On medical advisement, I had been taking 2 vegetable laxatives a day, and worried about the consequence of laxative dependency.

My cooking is now done exclusively in cast iron and glass. My aluminum pots and pans have been discarded. Since starting the diet I no longer require the use of a deodorant. When the chemicals in my body are being excreted through my pores, I do have a metallic body odor for 3 to 4 weeks duration. I've kept a couple sets of clothes aside for these "off weeks". Including miso in my diet is helping rid my body of heavy metals and thus decreasing chemical sensitivities. Decreasing these sensitivities has improved my memory, concentration, and comprehension. Poppy seeds are helping to purge nickle out of my body. Sulphur flower baths aid in pushing all the heavy metals out, as do seaweeds and ginsing root.

Working through the years as a registered nurse, I perceived my medical problems from my typical western training, which is, to treat the symptoms. Chronic sinusitis was treated frequently

with decongestants and analgesics. That medication
exposed me to phenol and corn, two ingredients that
are in numerous products, foods and chemicals. For
the same reasons, infections were treated with
antibiotics (often on a monthly basis from October
through May) which caused an overgrowth of Candida.
That, in me, caused irritability, psoriasis,
vaginitis, blurred vision, and cracking skin with
acute pain at the outer corner of each eye.

Miso, if started too early in the diet, will
cause the Candida to proliferate. I waited for my
counselor to advise me when to include miso in my
diet. My Candida is nearly completely under
control and I've completely cleared my psoriasis,
blurred vision and other eye symptoms.

I've learned that many foods that may not be
tolerated alone could be tolerated in combinations.
Millet, cooked with squash, and barley with rice,
are often tolerated in combination, if not alone.
When ingested by themselves, I became extremely
dizzy eating millet, and experienced muscle spasms
having barley. After cooking these combinations
for a period of time, my intolerance to them has
reduced and I can now tolerate them individually.

I've been told there is extreme heightened
sensitivity when the body is cleansing itself of
toxins. Many old symptoms are experienced such as
irritability and depression. An acute awareness of
this fact helped me keep the irritability in proper
perspective (at times...old patterns of behavior
are hard to break). The depression has completely
subsided except recently when a chemical overload
brought it on again. I reversed it with the use of
pressure points (acupressure), another health aid I
had learned.

The macrobiotic diet is not a simple thing. Foods cause the body to react in definite ways. While on vacation I couldn't eat my normal macrobiotic diet. I prepared whole grain rice to take with me for my meals and ate little else for 4 days. Being new to the diet and not knowing all the consequences, I hadn't realized that a full rice diet can bring on a major discharge of toxins. In those four days I developed sinusitis which took 6 months to bring under control. I've learned to treat sinus infections with ginger compresses, lotus root plasters and lotus root tea. It's a pleasure to have a treatment free of antibiotics and void of the subsequent Candida proliferation they produce.

Since becoming knowledgeable in the macrobiotic way, I've learned that moderation in all things leads to balance. I can choose to eat in balance, or out, and live with the consequences.

In my 9 months on the diet I have learned that what I eat can bring on old chronic symptoms, be they physical of mental. Macrobiotics taught me the role diet plays in effecting disease.

The diet alone is not the whole story. It takes an overall awareness of what works best for each individual and the effort to do it. I can't say enough for the power of positive thoughts and the belief that you can heal yourself. No one can do it for you. And medication is a questionable aid. I found a combination of advice from a number of holistic health professionals and extensive reading gave me the tools to decide what was best for healing me.

I began to understand that I had to reduce the bombardment of chemicals that I encountered daily. This saturation kept my sensitivities at such a high level my immune system didn't stand a chance of healing. I had to leave my job in a building that was full of toxins (for a chemically sensitive person). The toxins included fumes from paint, cleaning fluids, glue, hair sprays, perfumes, smoke, etc. My health started to improve significantly within two weeks of leaving the building. But on three return visits the severe symptoms recurred. It made me appreciate that I had made the right decision.

Rooms were continually being painted and the fumes circulated throughout the ventilating system into every room exposing everyone in the building. Often meetings would be held in rooms containing new carpeting. Out-gassing formaldehyde from the carpet, and phenol from the glue underneath, affected people to varying degrees. When meetings were held in the art room, we were exposed to paint supplies and plastic containers, each out-gassing phenol. Meetings held near the smokers' lounge left us with a prevalent smoke odor. Pesticide laden smoke from the smoking room carried into the rest of the building through the open hallway doors and ventilating system.

Even when I walked into an empty corridor, I was surprised to be overcome with lingering perfume odors from employees who had passed by earlier. I tried to control the pain and muscle spasms from these mysterious exposures through use of pressure points. But often the overload of toxins my body was encountering during the day was too great. I was left ill at the end of the day with acute muscle spasm pain, laryngitis, headache and nausea. These symptoms would clear after remaining 8 hours in my bedroom at home with my chemical filter. Seaweeds helped relieve me of chemical sensitivities and made me more tolerant of exposures to chemicals. I'm now more tolerant of exposures to chemicals, and when overloaded, clear faster of the symptoms they produce in me.

Another source of almost daily attack came from my neighbor's laundry. Whether clothes dried on the line or in a dryer, a heavy, perfumed odor was exhausted. The detergents used in the washing process and the fabric softeners all contained fragrances and often phenol. The normal wind direction from the west blows the phenol fumes directly toward our home. When the laundry is being dried, I must keep all windows closed, even on the warmest days, and cannot go outdoors to use my porch swing or tend to my gardening which I've always enjoyed. When one neighbor opens her front door, the chemical odor of the laundry soaps all but knocks me over. I wonder what hidden toll it's taking on that family's health since they will have breathed the phenol each day and night over a period of years?

I read that "the human body has an electromagnetic field that depends upon body energy being balanced". I became aware of energy imbalances and how to correct them when they occurred.

Acupuncture treatments helped me by dramatically reducing painful muscle spasms that were caused by exposure to chemicals and offending foods. I gained an understanding of the use of pressure points that the body has to allow me to control many symptoms of imbalance. I experienced ear aches when my kidneys were cleansing of toxins. This pain was relieved every day by a combination of aids using pressure points, ginger compresses to the kidneys twice a day, and 2 drops of warm sesame oil to each ear washed out with warm bancha tea containing sea salt. A happy added benefit is that antibiotics were not used and thus no Candida developed.

Yoga and deep breathing exercises have become part of my daily routine. Yoga has completely eliminated my chronic insomnia. I'm now asleep in 10 to 20 minutes, sleep through the night, and, thanks to the diet, awaken refreshed.

I've been told that meditation may be an integral part of the healing process and plan to implement this in the near future.

I discovered the discipline of macrobiotics extends beyond myself and relates to patterns of behavior and interactions within a family. I believe that my entire family will develop balance and harmony in their lives. Through an increased awareness of each other's feelings and thoughts, our psychological, as well as our physical beings are effected positively.

All this can seem overwhelming. It is a new approach to health. It consumes a considerable amount of time just to cook macrobiotically. My advice is to do as much as you can possibly do initially. Don't become frustrated because you're not able to do it all at once. Take each day to add as many new dimensions to your routine as you can.

In summary, macrobiotics has enabled me to develop a better understanding of how diet effects the way I feel physically and psychologically, to eat in balance, and in the process, to unload many chronic symptoms. It has also made me aware of other alternatives that are available. I now realize that my health will only continue to improve in the future with the use of this valuable approach.

The end result should be an understanding of how to bring order, balance, and harmony to your life. No one can ask for more.

by Kathryn M. Swatt, R.N.   5/30/88
with much support and help editing and arranging
from George F. Swatt, A.I.A.

I would like to thank Kathryn for sharing her macrobiotic experience with us. She reminds us of several good points:

(1) Lotus root is indeed good, especially for lung problems. The reason I hesitated in adding it was that it's difficult to find in a fresh form that is not moldy.

(2) The reason for failure to improve in a chemically sensitive individual may be that he has not reduced his chemical load sufficiently. Just as you would not ask a person who is trying to heal a wound macrobiotically to rub dirt into it each day, we cannot expect a diet to bring about healing in a system constantly bombarded by chemicals. If one has to leave work, it's advisable to first get proof of chemical hypersensitivity through testing in the office. Medical-legal proof is necessary for any form of disability.

(3) If one is interested in beginning to learn the type of physical diagnosis used by macrobiotic counselors, two beginning sources are Mishio Kushi's How to See Your Health: Book of Oriental Diagnosis and Natural Healing Through Macrobiotics, also Muramoto's Healing Ourselves.

D.J. was a 26 year old female with severe asthma and eczema over nearly her entire body. She improved with an ecologic program but her problems were compliance and money. If I could have taken her home with me and fed her and made her get her injections on time, she would have remained clear.

But she would cheat on the diet and not show up for her injections for months, then appear in tears. I recommended she learn macrobiotics. She returned to the office clear and happy, and it cost her far less than allergy treatments.

C.T. a 30 year old law student, had colitis that responded only partially to food injections and diet, but was markedly clearer on macrobiotics. After three years he modified his diet to include western foods and has remained good.

H.G. was a universal reactor, losing weight and a prisoner of her home. Within the first six months of macrobiotics she lost many of her chemical sensitivities and could venture out without a mask, gain weight, and in general felt markedly better.

The case examples mounted quickly as more people evaluated macrobiotics. Some made more rapid improvement by amalgam replacement. In general, most people who attempted macrobiotics were successful at improving their chemical tolerances.

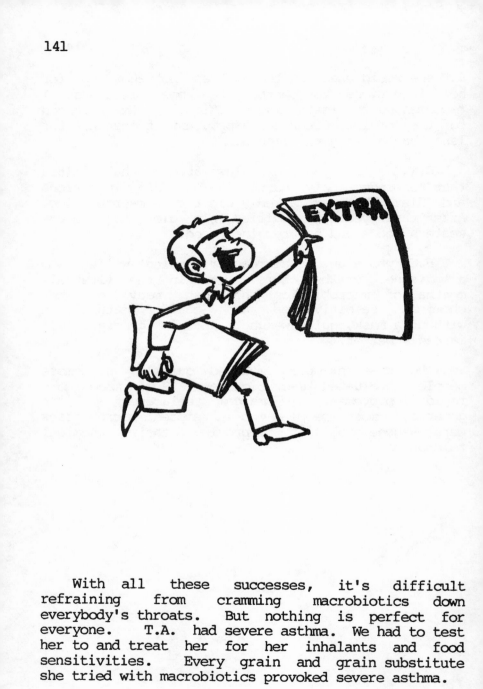

    With all these successes, it's difficult
refraining from cramming macrobiotics down
everybody's throats. But nothing is perfect for
everyone. T.A. had severe asthma. We had to test
her to and treat her for her inhalants and food
sensitivities. Every grain and grain substitute
she tried with macrobiotics provoked severe asthma.

CHAPTER VII

GEARING UP FOR THE TRANSITION

The Basic Four Food Groups

You and I all know from third grade that there are four major food groups. They used to make me feel really guilty at 8 years of age if my parents hadn't fed me something from all four groups for breakfast. Being the oldest (of eventually seven children), I had to help everyone else get ready and was lucky if I had a piece of toast or a bowl of Cheerios. Here they were telling me I should have:

dairy - milk
grains - toast
protein - eggs
fruits/vegetables - orange juice

That might work on Sunday, but never on school days. As I grew up and got out on my own, I found that the breakfast basic four could be quite delicious:

dairy - ice cream
grains - donuts
protein - left over steak
fruits/vegetables - chocolate
(you see chocolate comes from a bean, which makes
it a vegetable, I figured).

Then as I got sicker, in my thirties, I tried to eat more healthfully, so the breakfast basic four looked something like this:

dairy - 2 glasses of raw milk
grain - English muffin
protein - 2 eggs with 4 strips of bacon
fruits/vegetables - bananas

Then when I got into my health food kick, it transformed to:

dairy - yogurt
grains - granola
protein - nuts
fruits/vegetables - apples

When I became terribly allergic, the basic four went out the window. Breakfast might be four zuchini's one day and half a dozen shrimp the next.

___ ___ ___ ___ ___ ___ ___ ___ ___

MACROBIOTIC FOOD GROUPS

When I got started in macrobiotics, I was so overwhelmed by all the foods, I decided I had better devise a system to help me account for my newly found food groups. This is how I tally up each day:

Grains, Greens, and Beans
Seeds and Weeds
Roots and Fruits

Grains can be semi-rotated if need and can include (organic) brown rice, millet, or Hato barley. If intolerant, try quinoa, oats, amaranth, buckwheat, or rye. Grains will change with the stage of healing and season.

Greens include collards, kale, mustard greens, scallions, parsley, watercress, Brussel sprouts, but later can be broadened to romaine, endive, Napa cabbage, bok choy, and more.

% volume for each meal

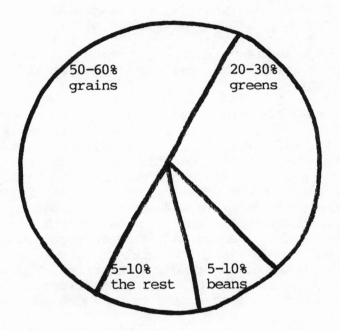

Try to make the volume of every meal about 50%
whole grains.

Beans can be azuki (aduki), garbanzo (chickpea), lentil, and lima, for starters.

Seeds and nuts can include sesame, pumpkin, and almond.

Weeds are the precious mineral-laden seaweeds; start with nori, arame, wakame, and hiziki.

Roots include carrots, onions, radishes, parsnips, leeks, turnips, and the medicinal burdock and daikon.

Fruits will only be "Fruits of the earth" for beginners: squashes. This includes all hard winter squashes and pumpkins. Cauliflower is also acceptable. I also considered fruits to mean "treats" and used that word to remind me to add the miso or tamari to my dishes, as it was indeed a real treat to tolerate a ferment and something with a real taste after two months of G, G + B. Other flavors (or "medicines", depending on your condition) could include grated ginger juice. Later a baked apple or pear or cherries, with steel cut oats once or twice a week may be allowed. More expansion and desserts appear as wellness occurs.

So for the first month, a quick meal can look like this:

spring water in saucepan
add diced carrots, onion, squash, and/or
    daikon.
steam a few minutes,
add chopped kale, collards, scallions,
    watercress, Italian parsley, mustard
    greens and/or dandelion.
place cold cooked brown rice or barley and
    beans on top,
cover and steam another couple minutes
DONE!

Now take inventory:

grains; yes, I choose organic brown rice today.
greens; yes, I'll have scallions and collards.
beans; yes, chickpeas.
seeds;- no. So sprinkle gomashio (an easy recipe
in most of the cookbooks) over the rice or make
sesame seed tea.
weeds;- no. I forgot the seaweeds, my wonderful
source of minerals. Add crumpled toasted nori
sheets or wakame. Or I could have cooked hiziki or
arame with the roots initially. Now where did we
leave off?

roots; yes, turnips from my organic garden
fruits - When tolerated, dissolve 1/2 tsp. chickpea
miso in a small aliquot of the steaming water.
Then add this back to the cooking pot and serve.
Some days I serve the rice with scallions in half
of a steamed acorn squash. Later you'll be able to
make yourself real desserts.

Now check the proportions:

Item	Generally Recommended %	Possible Range
grains	50%	30-65%
greens	25%	20-50%
beans	10%	0-15%
seeds	5%	0-5%
(sea)weeds	"	0-10%
roots	10%	0-10%
fruits	"	0-5%

You see, you don't need all the food groups
everyday. You don't need beans everyday, for
example. And you certainly would not want all the
choices in one group in one meal. For example,
prepare brown rice for 1-3 days, then cook

millet for variety for the next few days, then Hato
barley. If you are particularly rushed one day,
just make it 50-50, rice and veggies (greens,
cauliflower, squashes or roots). If you happen to
toss in some seaweed, all the better.

And when you get sophisticated you can separate
items into more elegant side dishes instead of
making one casserole-type meal. For example, you
could start with the roots and "fruits" in the form
of carrots in miso soup. Then make another side
dish of white baby lima beans in Kombu, another of
brown rice with toasted sesame seeds (gomashio),
and one of steamed kale. There you have a
macrobiotic meal with 4 dishes.

Congratulations: You have mastered one of the
most difficult transitions of going from an
American fast food diet into a healthful whole
grains and fresh vegetable macrobiotic diet. In a
few weeks, you will be on your way to a new level
of wellness. If it seems too extreme, you may be
happier with a more gradual transition. One option
is to merely reduce your portions of everything you
normally eat by 50%. Make up the difference in
brown rice and kale, 50-50. They will not taste
great, however, because your taste buds are being
bludgeoned by the extreme tastes of your regular
foods.

THE TRANSITION: <u>GO</u> <u>FOR</u> <u>IT</u>

The transition to macrobiotics can be done in many ways. You could start by cutting out sweets and meats, the two commonest extremes. So in order to have something to eat, you'd better slip in a whole, unbroken grain to every meal. So your first macrobiotic food will probably be organic brown rice. Try to work it up to 50% of each meal. Don't worry if you're not perfect - you're learning, so go easy on yourself. Next get some steamed greens into each meal and try for 25%.

Remember to chew very well. I used to bolt my food; one to three bites was usually max for me before I swallowed. But considering what I ate, it didn't require much chewing. When you eat whole grains, however, you should chew each mouthful until it is totally liquid. (1) It unloads your pancreas from unnecessary work, thereby helping your body heal hypoglycemia and other problems. (2) Saliva can actually change the food from acid to alkaline. (3) It increases and improves the amount of nutrients you get from the food.

Back to your transition, you could read Colbin's, <u>The</u> <u>Book</u> of <u>Whole</u> <u>Meals</u>. It not only has recipes but menus and preparation time schedules. Then just ease on into that transition; while phasing out sweets, meats, and dairy, phase in grains and greens. Hopefully from your E.I. experience you already are smart enough to be off processed foods. Ms. Colbin's book <u>Food</u> <u>and</u> <u>Healing</u> is excellent on theory.

Before macrobiotics I probably had beans and whole grains maybe once a year. I remember I made a barley soup once and had once cooked some brown rice just out of curiosity to see what the big deal was. Since neither one was as delicious (then!) as my sticky buns, I decided they took too long and were not worth the effort. So I left my beans to yearly picnics and decided to get my whole grains from oatmeal cookies!

Sadly, most of us totally ignore whole grains and beans and many greens. We actually had to learn how to cook brown rice, adukis and collards.

In the beginning you'll probably find it impossible to believe (as we all did) that your sweet craving can be controlled with sweet vegetables or balanced with sour (umeboshi). Or that your bitter craving (beer, coffee, cigarettes) will be controlled with bitter vegetables (endive, dandelion, escarole, chickory). But as you begin to get off the extremes of meats and sweets, and onto a more easily buffered whole grains and veggies diet, these extremes will no longer have as much appeal.

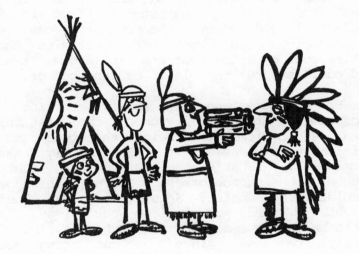

For starters, make a trade:

meats and sweets

for

grains and greens

Your first cooking priority is to start with grains and beans. What I do now is cook both two or three times a week so I have them ready for a couple of days to add to meals.

A word about washing grains: I thought it was silly to wash grains and beans -- after all you boil them! But by washing the grain you remove dust and dirt, fine stones (I've found some boulders!) and remove the rodent feces. Most importantly, you wash off mycotoxins that are toxins made by molds that are invisible, tasteless, and odorless, but capable of causing cancer.

So how does one go about starting on a macrobiotic program? Probably the first thing you need is commitment. Weigh the pros and cons critically to see if you really have the commitment. What's the worst thing that could happen with macrobiotics? First, there could be absolutely no benefit. Second, you may lose much weight. Third, you may lose your friends since you won't be eating meals at their houses, but that's easily remedied, since you can bring your own foods. Fourth, you will have to totally change your cooking, shopping and eating patterns and do a tremendous amount of reading, which will take time away from other activities. Fifth, if you don't go on a program appropriately with monitoring, you could make your symptoms worse and develop nutritional deficiencies. Sixth, you often have seaweed in your teeth.

And what's the best that can happen on macrobiotics? Obviously, you have a strong chance of clearing conditions that have resisted many other therapies and been termed incurable. You may arrive at new levels of health that you never dreamed possible.

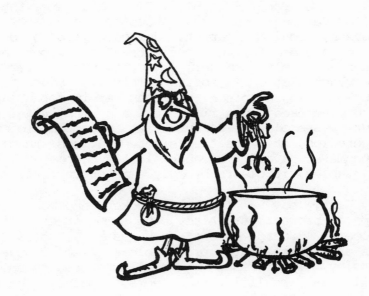

Some of the sights and smells will give you
second thoughts, but TRUST ME. Have I ever steered
you wrong?

How do you begin such an insurmountable task as starting a macrobiotic program? First, you should read the recommended books. In the meantime, go to the grocery store and buy some hard yellow or green winter squashes, such as acorn squashes, some large yellow onions, carrots, and scallions. Then go to an oriental market, (such as the Oriental House on Teall Ave. and Erie Blvd. E.) for a large fat root called daikon. Cut up a cup of each of these (squash, onion, carrot, daikon) into bite size pieces and add four cups of water to a pot and a pinch of salt and boil it for twenty minutes until the vegetables are soft. This is your "squash soup". In a pinch you can eat it for breakfast with precooked brown rice, or add the veggies to your casserole. Because it is composed of sweet vegetables, it helps the sweet cravings that many newcomers have. Because it is composed of sweet vegetables, it clears hypoglycemia pretty reliably.

Next, buy a pressure cooker and cook several cups of brown rice. Also, buy some greens at the grocery. Hard greens such as kale, collards, or mustard greens are preferable; also dandelion, parsley, watercress, or scallions can be used, as well as cauliflower, leeks, onion, parsnip, carrots, any hard winter pumpkins or squashes, Brussel sprouts, turnips and radishes. Napa cabbage or romaine lettuce would suffice if the other greens are not available. Also, purchase some assorted beans, such as chickpeas or garbanzo beans as well as aduki beans and perhaps some lentils and white lima beans. All the beans, grains, and specialty items can all be purchased by mail, through UPS, from Whole Earth Foods, 16 College Street, Clinton, New York, c/o Mr. Thomas Bell. Other local health food stores like Drumlins, (call collect 1-315-446-4820), Nottingham Road, Syracuse, NY, also carry most of these items and they can also be ordered from Mountain Ark

Trading Company, 1-800-643-8905, Fayetteville, Arkansas. In Syracuse at the University, there is also The Good Food Store, 316 Waverly Ave. in the Watson Theater Complex (315-423-3594), and Nature's Pantry on Erie Blvd., East. Most of these places will carry items you need if you only ask. I actually prefer to order by mail since it saves me time driving and shopping. Also the items come labelled when you shop by mail, and in the beginning most people don't know hiziki from wakame.

You can start out the first week rather simply. Put 1/2 cup of the squash soup liquid in a fry pan. Add some arame seaweed, which is an excellent source of minerals, to the veggie water and cook about two minutes. Then add the precooked rice just to heat it. You can add the precooked veggies here if any remain (or add new ones to the seaweed cooking cycle that preceded this since additional uncooked ones would require more cooking time). You can also cut up some of the kale or other greens and scallions and steam the whole thing in just two minutes. If more water is necessary, add it to this mixture. This can be eaten for breakfast, lunch, and dinner for the first couple of days or weeks until you start getting acclimated to the other foods and the recipes. There are many variations.

Until you get your bearings, you could exist on this a weak or more (I did, for over three months, as a trial). It's quick and easy to organize. Two or three times a week cook your squash drink, grains, and beans. When mealtime comes, first prepare everyone else's regular food. In the last minutes, cook your roots (onion, daikon, burdock, etc.), and seaweed in the squash soup juice or water for 5 minutes, add the precooked grains and beans and the chopped greens for another two to three minutes and you're ready to eat. The grains are warmed in the time the greens are steamed. Take inventory to see if you have included grains, greens and beans, weeds and seeds, roots and fruits. Sprinkle gomashio over the rice and mix in miso (and/or some ginger juice) if you can tolerate it yet. Check your proportions and serve.

Now if you can't manage that, you don't have a burning desire to get well; it's more like a flicker.

——— ——— ——— ——— ——— ——— ——— ——— ———

You will notice you are able to eat much larger amounts of foods than you ever did before and that you will start dropping weight. This is fine, because fat contains the foreign chemicals or xenobiotics, which need to be detoxified. You can put back the weight later on with good, clean organic foods.

You can use roasted barley tea as an in between drink, or once a week in the transition stage, some boiled almonds with the peels off. Simply squeeze them after they're been boiled for 10 minutes in water and they will pop out of their skins. Easy digestibility is an important factor and so is peace; each meal should be taken with a preliminary grace, expressing gratitude for the meal and good thoughts throughout the meal with very meticulous and thorough chewing. All foods and drinks must be well mixed with saliva to start breaking down the materials for proper digestion and assimilation.

In the evening you can add a half a cup or more of the beans, as well, to this mixture. You may be in a rush in the morning and choose to only have the squash soup or only the rice; then again you may have everything. You don't need beans at every meal or even every day. Substitute some vegetables like hard squash, cauliflower, or brussel sprouts.

You don't need greens at every meal. But these are good guidelines. Much depends on whether you are doing a transition diet (just getting used to whole foods and less meat, sweets, and dairy), a healing diet (which is the most strict of all), or a fun and creative maintenance diet (which can be masked "American" fare by talented cooks). Whichever, don't immerse yourself in guilt. There is no absolute right or wrong and learning is a commendable process.

Eventually you want to aim for at least 30 to 50% of each day's food and preferably each meal to be a whole grain, such as rice, oat, millet, barley, etc. It is best to start with rice the first week until you are sure of what other foods you should be having. If you're allergic to rice, try millet, corn, rye, oats, barley. Then try amaranth, quinoa (pronounced keen' wah), or buckwheat, since they are out of the grass family. If not successful, be sure they were organic before resorting to tapioca or no "grains" for a while. A consultation can provide further guidance.

At least 50% of the total diet should be vegetables. This includes greens, gourds (squashes) and root vegetables (turnips, carrots, onions, burdock, daikon), seaweeds, beans, nuts, and seeds as well as condiments and teas. Occasionally beer and sake are allowed after healing when a much broader diet is introduced. And some people really need red meat periodically after wellness has been attained. Nothing is cast in stone as evidenced by healthy specimens from all cultures. Many people need raw fruits and vegetables daily. There is much to be said for the life force which exists in living foods.

But if one is going to go on a program specifically for healing through macrobiotics, he should be resigned to the fact that most likely during the first six to twelve months he will not have any meats, sweets, processed foods, or fruits. If this type of commitment could not be made, I suggest the macrobiotic approach should not be considered.

There are other ways to deal with this, such as slowly introducing macrobiotic foods, but it appears that the cold turkey method is the best way to start to stomp out food cravings. Also, it's very difficult to appreciate the sweetness and goodness in many vegetables, such as carrots, turnips, onions and squashes when one is still eating honey, sugar, corn and cane sweeteners as well as artificial sweeteners. These strong sweeteners blunt the taste buds severely, or cause imbalances in the body chemistry, thereby maintaining cravings.

QUICK SUMMARY

(1) Stop meats, sweets, dairy. (This assumes you are health oriented enough to already have been off processed foods including alcohol and coffee.

(2) Begin 50-50 whole grains and vegetables.

(3) Further refine to grains, greens and beans, seeds and (sea)weeds, roots and "fruits". Watch that proportions are accurate.

Food Choices

Organization Begins with a List

Make copies of the following pages, right up to the Suggested Menu. Bring them to your consultation to check off what foods you can have. Then you have a ready made list to carry to the store for shopping as well.

In the meantime you will want to start making a list for your needs. From the grocery store you will need greens:

scallions	dandelion greens
mustard greens	parsley
kale	watercress
rappi	alfalfa sprouts
collard greens	Brussel sprouts

Grow alfalfa sprouts on your windowsill. Use cabbage or romaine if none of the above greens are available.

From the health food store you will need a good supply of medium grain brown rice, and you may want to have some short grain, as well. These can be rotated to avoid further sensitization.

medium grain brown rice
millet
rye
Hato barley

If you don't tolerate any of the above, try:

corn	amaranth
quinoa	buckwheat

(bulgar and couscous are wheat derived and somewhat processed, so avoid unless they are the only ones tolerated).

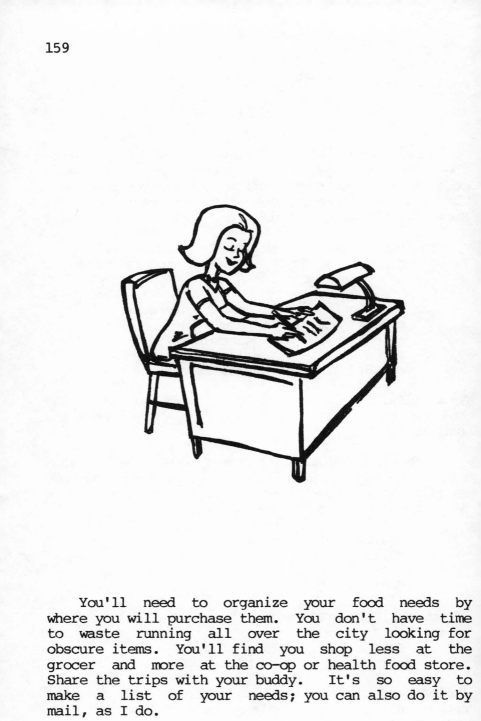

You'll need to organize your food needs by where you will purchase them. You don't have time to waste running all over the city looking for obscure items. You'll find you shop less at the grocer and more at the co-op or health food store. Share the trips with your buddy. It's so easy to make a list of your needs; you can also do it by mail, as I do.

Most of the vegetables can be obtained at the grocery except burdock, lotus and daikon, which are not always available, but Whole Earth Foods and the Oriental House often have some items.

Above Ground

cauliflower
hard winter squashes
cabbage
brussel sprouts
leeks

Below Ground

carrots (+tops)
onions (+ tops)
burdock root
lotus root
turnips
daikon (+ tops)
radish (+ tops)
parsnips(+tops)

Condiments:

umeboshi(plums) (very salty tasting but they can alkalinize you like alka-aid did for food and chemical reactions - See The E. I. Syndrome)
wheat-free tamari
chickpea miso
shitake mushrooms (one a week only)
ginger root (for compresses, tea, or flavoring)
thyme
scallions
sesame seeds (to make your gomashio)
wakame (for seaweed powder)
sage
sea salt

Beans:

| lentil | split pea | pinto | lima |
| azuki | chickpeas (garbanzo) | navy | mung |

Seaweeds:
nori   arame   kombu
wakame   hiziki

Oils:
Occasional olive or unrefined sesame (oils are usually not used in healing phase. Just stick to steaming until a consultation.)

Teas:
Bancha   Safflower
Roasted barley   Roasted rice
Sesame   spring water

Meat:
White fishes, including red snapper, halibut, shrimp, haddock, all with grated daikon/tamari (maximum twice a week in transition phase and wean to once every 2-4 weeks in healing phase, unless you need the calories and protein).

Sweets and snacks (Use very sparingly for healing; use only if you must, maximum once a week):

Yinnie rice syrup
Cooked fruits (apple, pear, cherries)
Chestnuts (available in late fall)
Rice cakes with tahini and yinnie syrup
Boiled, peeled almonds
Roasted pumpkin seeds with tamari
Mugwort mochi with daikon/tamari
Popcorn
Sunflower seeds

Cooking tools:

    Aeterum pressure cooker
    2   stainless steel sauce pans
    2   stainless steel fry pans
    1   good chef's knife
    1   good paring knife
    1   vegetable peeler
    2   collanders, large and medium
    1   bamboo tea strainer
    1   hand grater
    1   sushi mat
    1   spatula
    1   wooden spoon
    1   suribachi with pestle
    8   large glass storage jars for grains and
            seaweeds
    8   medium size glass storage jars for beans and
            nuts
    8   smaller size glass storage jars for teas,
            mushrooms and seeds
    2   wide mouth thermoses for work and travel
    1 or 2 covered, divided dishes for work and
            travel
    1   small picnic cooker for work and travel

Obviously you can't run out and get everything,
but work into your needs.   Also you may discover
many of these items at garage sales, for example.

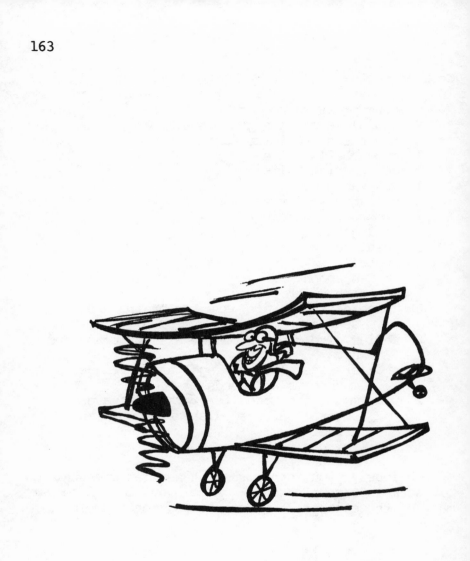

If it's a very long trip, order the vegetarian meals and pick at a dry salad and whatever else you can use. Bring along umeboshi-nori rolls and bottled water or bancha tea.

The following items may be allowed early, later on as a medicinal therapy, or not until you are better. You can bring this list to check off things that you could be having. Do not have them initially until you have had a consultation, but instead limit your diet to the items on the previous pages only.

Grains	Beans	Sea Vegetables
corn	kidney	agar-agar
wheat berries	Nato	dulse
(essene bread)	soy	Irish moss
noodles	tempeh	mekabu
flour products	tofu	

Vegetables	Fruits
broccoli	apples
cabbage	blueberries
celery	cherries
cucumber	grapes
endive	melons
escarole	peaches
green beans & peas	pears
Jerusalem artichokes	plums
kholrabi	raisins
mushrooms	strawberries
summer squashes	

Seeds	Teas	Meats
chestnuts	corsican	clams
sunflower seeds	dandelion	lobster
	kombu	white fish
	mu	(cod,flounder,
	nettle	halibut,sole,
		snapper)

Pickles and sauerkrauts

Sweets	Oils	Other
amazake	sesame	miso
apple juice	olive	shitake
barley malt	safflower	wheat-free soy
yinnie syrup		sauce
		horseradish
		lemon
		rice vinegar

Any other food that is not specifically listed in the earlier pages or circled on this list should be avoided until you determine your status at your next consultation.

In general, the healing phase requires reduction in beans, oils, and nuts. Avoid oats, salt, fish, spices, buckwheat, noodles, corn, raw salad, fruit, flour products or excessive liquids. Gomashio, umeboshi, miso and seaweeds plus at least twice weekly nishime cooking (using little water, see A. Kushi's <u>Cooking</u> <u>for</u> <u>Health:</u> <u>Allergies</u>), and ume sho kuzu (ibid) are helpful. But if you are having too many discharge symptoms, cut back particularly on miso and seaweed. Vary your cooking methods (steam, boil, bake, stir-fry, nishime and later raw); buy as organic as possible, do skin brushing.

Organization is easy if each time you enter the kitchen to prepare a meal, you simultaneously focus on the next 2 days or 6 meals. Organization is simple when you realize it's a tool of perspective or focus. Don't get so narrow that you only see the work of the meal before you. It could have been much easier at dinner time if you had, for example, cooked your rice while showering and having breakfast.

And each meal need not incorporate, as you see, the whole G., G. and B. scenario. That is to help you remember all the items you have available. As I prepare a meal and recite that, it reminds me to add the beans that I have hidden at the back of the refrigerator, or to add seaweeds at the beginning. It's to make life easier, not rigid. Breakfast can very well be left-over rice and bancha tea, only. Or it may be miso soup (with or with out any grains, greens, seaweeds, or roots.

If you ever find yourself in a panic asking "What can I eat?" Remember: When in doubt eat vegetables.

SUGGESTED MENU

For breakfast:

The squash drink with veggies and a bowl of
grains (add greens and gomascio if you have
time)

For lunch:

Take rice balls or nori rolls and steamed
greens and roots.

For dinner:

Grains, greens and beans, roots, sea vegetables
and squash as well as condiments. Do not eat
within 3 hours before bed, chew thoroughly.

Teas may be taken throughout the day, but in
general limit your intake unless you are thirsty.
If very thirsty, rinse the salt from the seaweeds
or cut back on miso.

Adjuncts:

breathing exercises
yoga
spiritual re-assessment
skin brushing
shiatsu or other body
    work
meditation
gratitude

positive imagery
herbal baths and
    compresses
therapeutic touch
phenolics
electro balancing
acupuncture, acupressure

Practice makes everything easier. Consult the
cookbooks when you're bored and ready to grow. And
remember there is no right or wrong, merely a
relentless quest for improvement.

You'll feel the need for condiments eventually.
Most are made with miso, soy or tamari sauce and

are in Esko's two cookbooks. Besides, gomashio to sprinkle on rice or grains, you can make sea vegetable powders early on when you can't yet tolerate the ferments. They are also rich in minerals. Simply roast kombu or wakame, for example, in the oven at 350 degrees until crisp, but not burned. Grind in suribachi and serve. Also they can be mixed with the gomashio.

Onion butter or carrot butter would be good for lunches as a spread. Put 1 tsp sesame oil in a pot, add 10 diced onions (or carrots), saute 5 minutes until translucent. Add a pinch of salt and just enough water to cover, cook on low a few hours until dark and sweet. You may need to add occasional water.

Chickpea dip or spread can be made in a variety of ways, as can many vegetable dips. Cooked beans can be pureed with finely diced onion, parsley and pitted umeboshi (plums). Or for hummus, add tahini (1:8 ratio, tahini to chickpea), garlic, lemon juice, parsley and a pinch of salt.

If your grains or beans become dull, cook them with kombu (acts like MSG as flavor enhancer) or onions. Don't be afraid to experiment once you know your temporary for limitations and have read a couple of cookbooks for a basic feel.

Lunch no longer needs to be limited to grains and greens, or nori rolls or stew. You could lightly steam vegetables (keep them crisp) and make a bean dip (water-sauteed onions, masked with beans, sesame and garlic. This could contain herbs, oil, other veggies, seeds, etc. as desired or allowed.). You can create bean or vegetable pates (use millet "bread" as vehicle).

If you're too strapped for work lunch ideas, don't push yourself. Slide backwards into a transition diet and use rice bread (yeast free), blue organic corn chips, essene bread or rice cakes for a while.

Note MB = Macrobiotic

Diet Sustitution Stages

Avoid (Standard diet)	Transition (not MB, but getting there slowly)	Healing (restricted temporarily until you are well)	Maintenance (includes all healing foods)
white bread	rice cake	organic brown rice	MB breads, pastas, grains
French fries	organic corn chips	barley, millet, ltd. oats	corn, soy, etc.
cheese	yogurt	seaweeds	tofu
coffee	herb tea	bancha tea	many MB teas
meat	fish fowl	beans	tempeh, fish
sweets/ snacks	fruits	squash drinks, pumpkin seeds, boiled, peeled almonds	see MB dessert bks fresh fruit popcorn
sandwich	yeast free rice bread, sprouts avocado	nori roll, millet "bread" vegetable spreads	cabbage rolls, MB breads + spreads

Avoid	Transition	Healing	Maintenance
Iceberg lettuce/ tomato salad	romaine, all veggies	steamed kale collards, onion, daikon, carrot, squash, Brussel sprouts, lotus root, parsley, watercress, dandelion, carrot tops, scallions,	pressed or raw salads, blanched veggies
ketchup, mustard, mayo, Hollandaise		gomashio, chickpea miso, wheat free tamari, ginger, garlic	herbs,MB pickles, sauces, dressings, olive + sesame oil
cream sauce		kuzu	tofu, kuzu + agar-agar sauces
processed frozen canned	fresh	organic	organic

You see from the above that there are 3 ways to center a MB healing diet:
    (1)   jump in
    (2)   ease yourself in via a transition
    (3)   ease yourself in via MB
           maintenance diet.

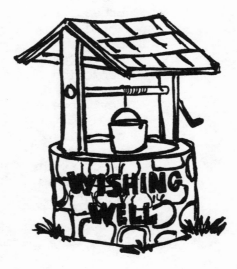

At this point, if you're wishing you had never picked up this book, maybe you're not committed enough to your health at this time.

However, if you're wishing you could hire a macrobiotic cook, then keep going -- you'll get there, without one.

Getting Further Organized

Tools you will need to purchase right away are a good pressure cooker (Aerturnum is a good model with safety features so it's less likely to explode in your face), a strainer, a chef's knife as well as paring knife, sprouting jar and an assortment of at least three stainless steel frying or boiling pans, with covers, large and small colander, tea strainer, a grater, and a mortar (and pestle) called a surinami (and surikogi).

Also, you'll want large gallon size glass jars to store the grains, beans, and seaweeds and smaller ones in which to store the teas. Remember grains need very dry storage or mycotoxins can result.

At this point you're wondering about backing out. I know, because I went through this for several weeks, wondering if I were doing the right thing. The foods were so strange, some of them smelled like swamp water. The recipes looked terribly uninviting and some of the compresses that I was instructed to use were so bizarre I was hysterical with laughter. You must be sure to leave time each day to do some yoga exercises and skin brushing. These stimulate the circulation. Meditation is also important.

So let's regroup - you now have bags all over the kitchen of strange looking things that you're not exactly eager to eat. First, you need to organize:

(1) Clean out your cupboards. Get glass containers and group beans, then grains, then teas, then sea vegetables.

(2) Cut up veggies for squash soup and start cooking.

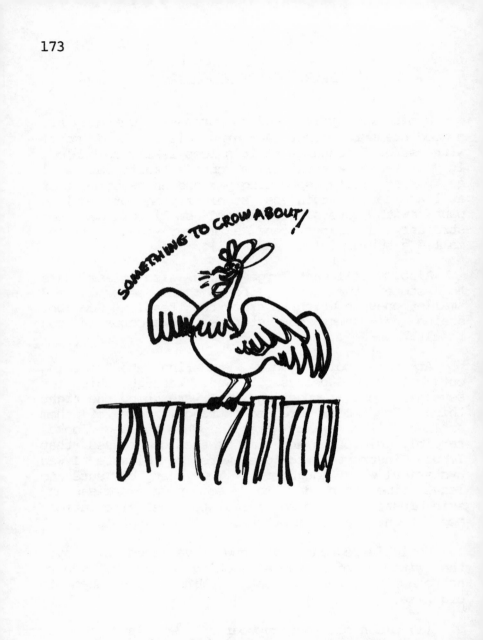

Hey, you're doing great, You can make squash soup, brown rice, greens, beans and miso soup.

(3) Cook up some brown rice.

(4) steam some kale or collards.

(5) Soak kombu and chickpeas to cook later or tomorrow.

(6) Give yourself a pat on the back, you've really accomplished a great deal.

At mealtime, just remember these rules:

(1) "Grains, greens, and beans".
If you must omit something, make it the beans. 50-50, 30-70, or 60-40% are all acceptable ratios of whole grains to vegetables depending upon your condition. 50-50 is safer for starting if you have not yet had a consultation. And if you tolerate no grains, it's obvious: eat veggies for awhile. You may require even further modification.

(2) If in the beginning the formula seems too difficult, temporarily consider that "Greens" could really mean all vegetables in general, in which case they could be 35-65% (preferably 45-55% of each meal). Each day try to get these five types of vegetables: greens or green vegetables (either kale, collard, mustard, dandelion, parsley, watercress, scallions, romaine, etc), above ground veggies (squash, cauliflower), below ground or root veggies (turnip, burdock, onion, carrot, daikon), sea veggies (hiziki, wakame, arami, kombu, nori), and dangling veggies or beans (lentils, chickpea, lima, azuki).

(3) After a few months, or as soon as you tolerate it, get some ferments each day (miso, tamari) and pickles.

(4) Watch your overall percentages. In the first few months beans should be only a couple times a week for allergic people. Then when they become daily, never should they be more than 15% of a meal. Likewise, seaweed should constitute 5-15% of a meal.

(5) At each meal be sure to check if you need to have something soaking (beans, seaweed), cooking (grains or beans),or sprouting (alfalfa) for the next day.

A note about chewing: Each mouthful should be chewed at least 50 times. You are eating 50% starch and the digestion of starch begins in the mouth with the admixture with saliva.

So to re-iterate, when breakfast rolls around, you could eat your precooked squash soup, add your rice and beans, top it off with a couple of sheets of crumpled, toasted nori (hold over high flame until it turns green) and add diced collard greens and scallions. Cover 5 minutes while steaming. Put some miso in a bowl, add some of the cooking water to dissolve it; add the dissolved miso to the soup and mix. You are ready to serve. I've repeated this intentionally, since this seems to be the commonest stumbling block. Macrobiotics is not just a diet, but getting into the diet is the most difficult part for most.

You could get a hot plate at work and a teapot for midmorning and afternoon. Occasional boiled almonds, daily nori rolls, occasional mugwort mochi and grated daikon and tamari could be a snack. For lunch you could bring more of breakfast. By dinner

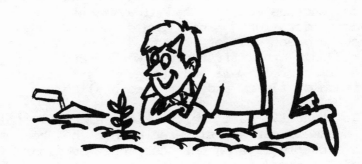

Start an organic garden

(1) it is good exercise
(2) it gets you out in the fresh air
(3) it's satisfying to watch things grow
(4) it will provide you with inexpensive organic
produce

time and weekends you'll start exploring the recipe books or have your same basic meal, perhaps just varying it with different seaweed, grains, beans, and veggies. The concepts are balance at each meal. Watch your percentages -- on the average, grains 50%, greens 25%, and all else falls in the remaining slot (beans, seeds and seaweeds, roots and "fruits").

You can vary the ingredients or even rotate. You will eventually get into other menus, but I had personally lived this way for three months. I was never hungry. I did have to work at keeping 120 pounds, whereas before I had always been 10 or 15 pounds overweight and could never budge them without a great deal of effort. They slipped off effortlessly the first two weeks and during the whole time I felt well and satiated and didn't get my afternoon slump, and I started healing.

For travel, nori rolls with umeboshi (plums) and steamed carrot slivers cannot be beat. You could actually live on this for three or four days. Boiled almonds and steamed vegetables with beans and grains can also be made up ahead of time for travel. Bring some dry roasted pumpkin seeds, too. You could make steamed leaves rolled about grains for travel (similar to cabbage rolls, only you'll use steamed kale or collards).

For dining out, stuffed squash and nori rolls, available at the Cafe Margeaux, James Street, can be ordered ahead to take to other restaurants. You can also add a dish of steamed greens. When you're out in other restaurants, order a small portion of fish, and a large double portion of steamed vegetables. You can decide if you want raw salad without dressing and their bleached white rice or not. I like to sneak nori rolls into my pocket and let them magically appear on my plate. This balances the rest. And remember attitude, a sense of humor and enthusiasm for wellness are crucial.

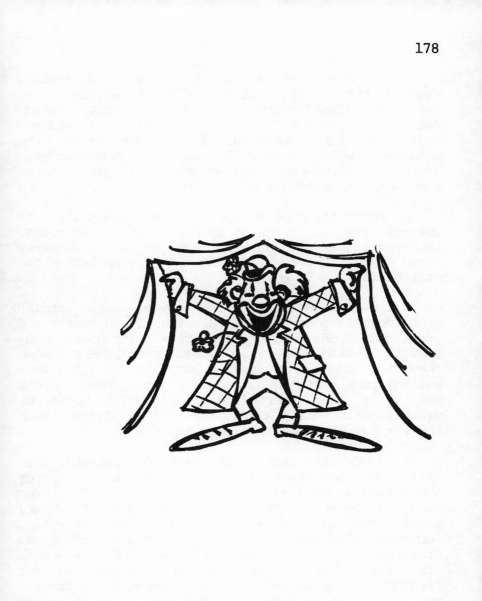

Are we having fun yet?

Each person would benefit from a counseling session for their specific condition and follow up is crucial since living organisms are not static. You will change, and your needs will change. Regardless of how great you feel at any point, the pendulum will eventually swing. Remember the difference between corrective and maintenance levels for nutritional corrections?

A corrective prescription was necessary to correct you but if kept up beyond the corrections, you created new imbalances. And so a maintenance level was needed. The same applies for macrobiotics.

Remember back to the people with Candida problems? As soon as they eliminated ferments and processed foods and sugars from their diets, many started feeling wonderful and had more energy than they had had in years? But because they were eating such an unbalanced, high meat diet, eventually they started going downhill months or years later. This is because the pendulum swung too far in the opposite direction.

They present with the classic problems that tell you they are eating out of balance. (1) They don't feel as good as they did before. (2) They need to be very strict, for if they cheat they feel awful, and (3) they have terrible cravings. Conventional medicine has no concept of this. Cravings are a symptom of imbalance. Dietary needs are not static. Good balance is crucial for constant wellness, and periodic assessment assures we are eating at the fulcrum. Even eating macrobiotically requires assessment due to your changing needs and seasons.

Follow-up Questionnaire

Periodic assessment is crucial for success. Before each follow-up consultation copy and fill out the following questionnaire. In this way you will be able to concentrate on your real needs and not get lost in the details of daily living. Bring this completed form to each follow-up visit. Many will want to copy the first version and merely add to it for subsequent visits with different colored ink.

_____

Name_____

Date_____

How long have you been practicing macrobiotics?____

What were your primary six symptoms and reasons for doing so?_____
_____
_____
_____
_____
_____
_____

What have you accomplished thus far?
_____
_____
_____
_____
_____

What remains to be accomplished?

_____

_____

Have you had any discharges? _____ How many? _____
Describe the most pertinent:

_____

_____

_____

_____

_____

Were blood tests done for any of these? _____

What are 4 average breakfasts like?

(1) _____

_____

(2) _____

_____

(3) _____

_____

(4) _____

_____

4 lunches?

(1) _____

_____

(2) _____

_____

(3) _____

_____

(4) _____

_____

4 dinners?

(1) _____

_____

(2) _____

_____

(3) _____

_____

(4) _____

_____

4 snacks?

(1) _____

_____

(2) _____

_____

(3) _____

_____

(4) _____

_____

What are your general percentages like?

_____
_____

When were your nutrient (vitamin, mineral, etc.)
levels last checked? _____

What adjuncts have you evaluated, duration and
    results? _____
_____
_____
_____

What MB books have you read?

_____

_____

_____

_____

_____

How much weight have you lost?_____

    Check the percent improvement you experienced during the following intervals since starting macrobiotics:

	Worse	25% better	50%	75%	100%
1st month					
2nd month					
3rd month					
4th month					
5th month					
6th month					
other					
1 year					
2 years					
other					

Overall, what is your assessment of macrobiotics for you?_____

_____

_____

_____

What are its drawbacks for you?

_____
_____
_____

What would make MB easier for you?

_____
_____
_____

Other comments:

_____
_____
_____
_____
_____
_____
_____
_____

Are you using any injections, supplements or
    medicine?_____
_____
_____

Are you using any herbs?_____
_____

Besides the diet, what else are you doing for
    yourself?_____
_____
_____
_____
_____

How much exercise do you get?

_____
_____
_____

185

What is the problem for which you have come for today?

_____
_____
_____
_____
_____
_____
_____
_____
_____
_____
_____
_____
_____
_____
_____
_____

Have you consulted a counselor?
   Who _____
   When _____
   Advice _____
         _____
         _____
   Result _____
         _____
         _____
         _____

Are You Feeling Overwhelmed?

You should be. You're making a major lifestyle change so you can determine if macrobiotics feels right for you. And because of individual biochemistry no one can give a blanket diet that would fit everyone. But we can give you a general overview that could be modified or adapted to the needs of many. If you don't fit into this scheme, you'll need an individual consultation. Whether or not you need it initially, you should have one within the first three months to check many aspects of your program to optimize your quest for wellness.

As with the Candida and rotation diets, this entails much work on your part. Reading, studying and practice are necessary. More important are the psychological blocks that a person unknowingly thwarts his own efforts with. Because of all of these factors, more than ever we must make it clear that the phone is not the place to bargain for foods or to go over your diet questions. Do not call the office regarding your diet. Reread this book.

If you're having a bad reaction, schedule immediately. If you think you are merely discharging, get a blood test only. If you have a few well-thought out questions that require short answers, print or type them double spaced on a large paper with enough room after each question for a reply. Include a self-addressed stamped envelope.

———— ———— ———— ———— ———— ————

A logical beginning is to learn to cook organic brown rice and steam kale. Substitute if food intolerances exist. You could live on this a few days as you slowly introduce squashes, carrots, onions and other greens. Next begin to learn to cook beans so that within the first 1-3 weeks you have grains, greens and beans. You should get your seaweeds, roots and seeds (gomashio is a good first item or roasted pumpkin seeds) in during that time. Miso may not be tolerated until after several months, but periodically (every 2 weeks) give it a try.

Your meals can have many formats: the casserole method described combines everything in one bowl. Or you can separate things as individual dishes. As you begin to add other grains and greens, veggies, and seaweeds, you can even rotate if desired.

You can vary your cooking style as well: pressure cooking, steaming, stir-fry with water, baking, etc.

Stuffed squash, nori rolls, casseroles, and individual dishes having been accomplished, you'll be ready to devour the cookbooks for ideas. You'll even come up with handy ideas that are not in the most popular books. For example, millet cooked in the same grain/water proportions as rice (2:3) in a pressure cooker for 40 minutes comes out like a firm bread. It's so firm it can be sliced and used as a vehicle for many spreads like mashed beans or veggies. Later on when you can have oil it can be sliced and sauteed like tofu. There are many sauces that can be added, like a green sauce of scallions and kuzu. For larger slices, cook millet in a covered saucepan and firmly press it while it's hot into a loaf pan. Slice when cool.

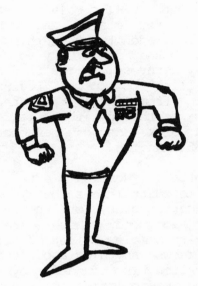

Don't be too tough a task master on yourself. You can only do what you can do. You'll eventually reach your goal if you are determined enough.

Attitude

Obviously if you thought the four day rotation diet was impossible, or even just the rare food diet, you should not attempt macrobiotics. Also, it should be quite evident that if you do not have cooperation, approval, and loving help from a spouse and relatives, your chances at success are minimal and it will only create tremendous friction. If you moaned and groaned your way through rotation, don't even think of attempting macrobiotics. And don't try to cram macrobiotics down everybody's throat. You're the one who is sick and willing to do it. Loving support is all you can expect from family. Rarely will anyone benefit from a therapy that is forced upon them. When one is sick enough, perspectives have an amazing way of changing.

People often question after they've read something like Sattilaro's book, "Why doesn't the American Cancer Society or the American Medical Association recommend these treatments?" The reasons are very simple. First of all, it's a rare doctor who knows anything about them. Much of our medical education is funded by pharmaceutical companies and macrobiotics does not make any money for them. Second of all, many people will not follow up and consult with the physician, so that he does not keep learning from seeing hundreds of people struggle through these conditions. There is a need for documented studies, but instead people go off and do it, never teaching us about it. If a doctor saw several patients a week who were steadily improving resistant conditions with MB, he'd get very interested. Third, most people would just plain not do it; even some people with cancer would not be able to change their lifestyles to the extent that macrobiotics requires. So, by all means save yourself a great deal of aggravation and

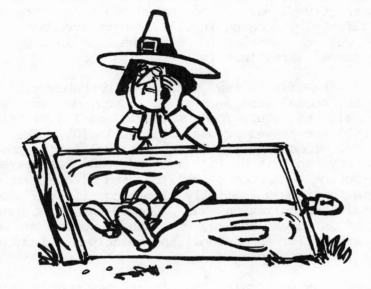

If you feel that your social life is cramped because of macro, you need an attitude and organizational reassessment. Call your macro buddy for help with a creative solution.

possibly even a divorce by not even attempting it,
unless you have made a commitment to yourself to
take a couple of years out of your life to devote
to the pursuit of a new level of wellness.

If you think you can quietly factor it into
your lifestyle without anyone else knowing, think
again. You must be prepared for all of your friends
and relatives having to make adjustments to your
new lifestyle, because it will involve everyone in
some way or another. Everyone that is a part of
your normal life, that is.

In the first few months you probably will not
have any social engagements, or if you do you will
take all of your food with you, as I did. Also,
you will not travel or you will, as I did, take all
of your food and cook it. A travel picnic cooler
is a very handy item to have as well as several
wide-mouthed thermoses and covered dishes. It can
become extremely socially limiting if you don't
maintain organization and a good sense of humor.
Many of us cook double, in other words we make
regular meals for friends and relatives and our own
meals for ourselves.

Not having fruit the first few months is not
easy as well and the smells of some of the seaweeds
cooking have been described as "low tide", and
that's being courteous. When your whole house
smells like this, it makes you have second
thoughts. You may spend two to three hours (if
you're not organized) cooking and cutting each day.
You will need to plan your meals and your time much
more carefully than you ever did before, and it's
not just a diet change; it's a lifestyle and
attitude change. There is more to improved health
through macrobiotics than can be put in one book.
It is not merely a diet.

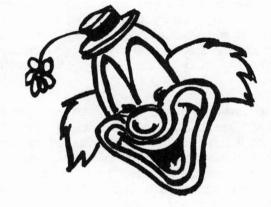

As with all of life, a sense of humor is most useful. How can you flood yourself with damaging emotions like anger, frustration, and depression when you're laughing.

But in spite of all this, macrobiotics makes so much sense biochemically, and it has such a remarkable track record, that it certainly seems worth a try for many who have nowhere else to go. But I must stress from the outset that, if you're going to be the least bit depressed, or complain one iota about it, you probably will not make it and you shouldn't even attempt it. Fortunately for most of us, we started feeling so good, so clearheaded and so much more level in terms of emotions, and we started having so many symptoms melt away, that we were able to maintain an optimistic attitude and sense of humor. Never once did we have to get angry or militant or defensive. Nor did we have to get on our little soap boxes and start teaching everyone. This is the type of attitude that you must have; if you don't think you can handle it, don't even try. When you're ready you'll know, and when you hurt enough, nothing is impossible.

While making one of my fuzzy seaweed medicinal teas, that smelled like low tide at Nantucket, I began thinking how important a sense of humor is for enabling one to adapt to this new lifestyle. I thought maybe that was how people were cured of cancer through macrobiotics. They actually laughed so much that they spurred the immune system to new heights of adaptability (ala Norm Cousins).

Meanwhile, in a matter of weeks, strange smells were filling the house. Bags of black and green seaweeds greeted me in the pantry. My nails and knuckles had been grated down to a stage of blood and bones as I was learning to grate daikon and ginger. What remained of my hands was nearly burned off while toasting my nori sheets. I had yellow teeth from my safflower tea, a sunken chest and face from my weight loss and scars on my wrists and fingertips from trying to cut through rocky hard squashes.

I had burned so many grains in learning to use the pressure cooker, that I was on a first name basis with the fire department. Our smoke alarm became the dinner bell. But I can honestly say, through it all I enjoyed every minute and found lots to laugh about. The thing is I felt so much better than I had in years and here I had already thought that I had arrived; that I could feel no better. For indeed through ecologic management, I had attained such undreamed of levels of wellness, that I dared not hope for any more.

Just think how much simpler this whole experiment in health would be if you could choose a macrobiotic selection in any restaurant or airplane. That day may come.

Attitude and especially a sense of humor and a loving spouse, are beyond a doubt the primary ingredients to this program. The nuts and bolts you can get from reading and studying and you will have to do a great deal. What we provide here is rationale, motivation, and an organizational guideline to help you get started. You will need to come in for counseling and/or referral to suit your individual needs if you are going to try to maximize your program.

This book was written in an attempt to bridge the gap and ease the transition for you. You will get maximum benefit from it if you highlight and mark pages liberally for your own reference and review.

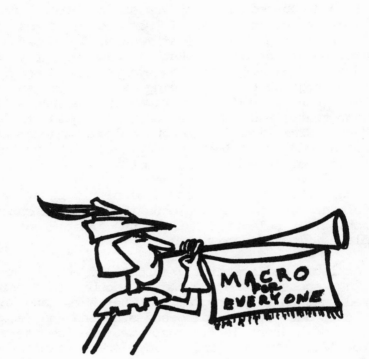

Try to resist converting everyone.
If they're interested, they'll ask you.

How To Make Maximum Use Of This Manual

(1) Start on the diet. If you have questions, do
not call the office, except to schedule a
consultation. We will see you any time you
need. If there are questions reread the manual
and also read the other recommended books. You
are too individual for phone communication and
relayed messages; they do not accomplish nearly
as much as a one-to-one confrontation. They
just allow you to slide into dependency and not
read. And as they do not allow for in depth
dialogue, the answers and conclusions may be
erroneous. For every question you ask, we
may have six questions that we need the answers
to in order to provide you with the best
solution. However, if you're fairly certain
your questions are straight-forward and require
no interaction, write them up as described and
send them in with a self-addressed envelope.

(2) For your first consultation, bring a copy of
the Diet Questionnaire (pages 90-97) and have
it filled out before your visit. Also bring a
copy of Food Choices (pages 158-165).

(3) Once you have started the diet, always bring a
copy of Food Choices and the Follow-up
Questionnaire (pages 180-185). After you have
filled it out the first time (having been on
the diet at least one month), you can make
extra copies of it and merely add to it using
different colored ink to update it for
subsequent visits.

Having your questionnaires ready saves a great
deal of time. Instead of asking you all these
questions and waiting for you to formulate your
reply, we can get on with the more creative
aspects of your individual program.

CHAPTER VIII

WHERE'S THE BEEF?   QUESTIONS AND ANSWERS

Q. What is macrobiotics?

A. Macrobiotics is a way of life that attempts to
harmonize with nature and not fight nature or
drastically alter her while adapting to modern
technology. Macrobiotics recognizes that a
person's health is foremost determined by what
he eats, but also by how he eats and cooks, as
well as his thoughts and his surroundings. It
extends to all levels of a person from his
individual person to his family, friends,
community, nation, and world, and his
relationship with all of these.

Q. My spouse doesn't want anything to do with
this. Shall I just go ahead anyway?

A. As with E.I., love and support of your spouse
are crucial. I can't tell you how my heart
soured when my husband repeatedly insisted
that I just do what I had to do. I wrestled
with the guilt for a long time and vacillated,
cooking him "regular" meals, then, "healthy",
and then macro (none of which I do well). He
was and is an absolute saint. Don't think
it's easy - I was still wrestling with guilt
in the fifth month and he lost over 30 lbs!
You'll need to experiment with what's best for
you. Love conquers all.

Q. How far do I need to go? Do I have to learn
all that yin and yang business?

A. That is an excellent question and I do not
have an answer. Having read widely on macro
and talked with many "converts", I have mixed
feelings. As with any endeavor there are

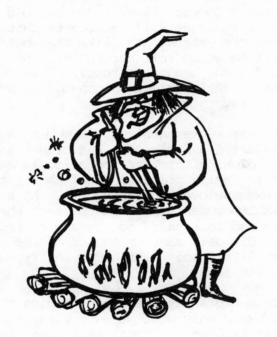

Macrobiotics is not a cult, not a religion, not a form of sorcery. It merely is a way of life that attempts to harmonize with nature.

those who feel it's an all or nothing phenomenon. But if one studies macrobiotics, you see wife beating, for example, is advocated. I sloughed this point off, thinking it had obviously changed since it was an old out of print book on macro philosophy. Then I read the 1988 Macromuse issue which featured George Ohsawa's 90 year old widow, and learned she still advocates this. There were other statements, like she would work until he would tell her to rest (not until she decided she needed to rest). This negates the concept of individual biochemistry for starters.

In other works hairiness in women is considered a bad sign. But oriental women, regardless of diet are notoriously non-hairy and in family practice I had the opportunity to examine over 10,000 bodies. At a macro talk two women supported the fact that indeed they had less hair, but they were ironically both blonde: another sector of the populous with little body hair. But the French or Italian lass?

Some macro's may feel we're raping their name and using only what we want without understanding the total philosophy (much of which is quite beautiful, actually). In that case, I made a mistake by giving credit to the source of my ideas. I should have pilfered what I could use and taught it under the guise of a modification of the rare food diet (see The E.I. Syndrome). For that is indeed what it is. It's a whole foods, peasant type of eating, devoid of commonly ingested antigens. There is no milk, wheat, eggs, corn, citrus, coffee, chocolate, beef, sugar or processed foods. And it does pay attention to biochemical balance better than any other diets I have encountered.

But I have chosen not to do that, and to promote macrobiotics as a modality for healing for people who have exhausted everything else. Clearly there are, however, stages or levels of involvement in macrobiotics and many may never choose to or need to become total converts in order to benefit.

The yin/yang as the Chinese knew it was reversed by Mr. Oshawa years ago. Then when foods are cooked a certain way they are said to become more yin or yang. Even long-time macrobiotic people cannot agree on whether a specific food is yin or yang. And since there is no proof and no yin/yang meter, this business discourage many who could have benefitted from the rest of macrobiotics.

As you'll see in the next chapter, learning acid and alkaline and yin and yang is important to your success in being able to balance yourself. But no diet is perfect. Critics argue that macro is too high in salt, too low in precious oils (that govern the integrity of all cell membranes, for one), low in B12, too rigid, too unadaptable for western man, etc. But these items can all be monitored and overcome.

Q. How do I select a macrobiotic counselor?
A. We are constantly evaluating them for their effectiveness with patients. When I called the Kushi Institute, I learned there are four levels of certification. There are no counselors within a 200 mile radius of the office who have the top three levels of certification. We attempt to match each person with the best counselor for them. That is why we insist if you want us to be part of your care, you should send us a copy of a tape recording of your session with your counselor.

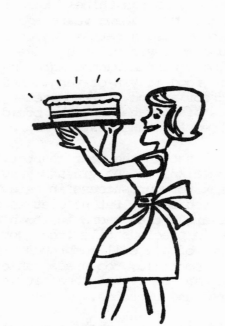

If you're still having cravings, you're eating out of balance. Don't suffer; let's find out what's wrong.

However, remember that many people in the diagnostic mode, and that includes macrobiotic counselors as well as doctors, get easily hung up in one area. You all know there are some doctors who do environmental medicine who think every patient has Candida or every patient has to get rid of the gas in their homes, and likewise there are macrobiotic counselors who are familiar only with the old standard diagnoses of heart disease, cancers, arthritis, et cetera. They are not aware of the problems and intricacies of E.I. They have probably never seen such profound nutrient deficiencies as we have documented in patients with E.I., and they are probably not aware that many of us have sequestered many chemicals which may take years to depurate or detoxify; and this may retard our healing immensely. Healing can likewise be retarded indefinitely in a too chemically contaminated environment for that individual. We will recommend the best counselor for your condition that we can. Again, it's a tailor made decision and some people need no counselor.

I saw two different "counselors" and their diagnoses were 180 degrees out of phase. Two excellent books for starters would be Acid and Alkaline (Herman Aihara) and Food and Healing (Anne Marie Colbin).

Q. Why is meat so bad?
A. In older days, a festival or feast was a rare occasion for celebration. All the stops were pulled as the banquet tables were prepared. Now we are such an affluent society that we have a feast everyday. Not only is a diet high in amino acids too acidic for many (requiring too much buffering), but on a

worldwide view it makes even less sense. It
takes 30 times more grain to raise a beef,
compared with the number of people that you
could feed with that grain. In addition the
animal concentrates pesticides many fold. But
the immediate problem is with its high
acidity. You know, for example, someone with
serious liver or kidney disease must restrict
his protein, whereas his grains are
sustaining. This is because in his weakened
condition some of the buffering mechanisms are
already malfunctioning. Why stress our bodies
unnecessarily on a day to day basis and over
work our marginally operating buffer systems?
Save it for a feast or special occasion.

Q. How do I know if I'm getting enough calcium if
    I'm not drinking milk?
A. You can get just as much, if not more, calcium
    from an equivalent amount of greens such as
    collards, kale, and watercress, also almonds,
    and many other foods. Colbin's Food and
    Healing, and Aihara's Basic Macrobiotics
    are some of the many books that will give
    equivalents of many of the nutrients and
    nutrient values of many of the foods.
    Remember when we lectured in China for a month
    in 1985, we never had or saw any milk or
    cheese, and they do not have nearly the
    osteoporosis incidence that we do in this
    country. One, we're not big greens eaters,
    and two, most of our foods are processed which
    means they have high levels of phosphates
    which inhibit the absorption of calcium. So we
    have two major mistakes. Next, high acid
    (meat and sugar) diets pull calcium out of
    bones to buffer the acid. Also calcium
    absorption depends on proper stomach acid and
    accessory minerals (boron, magnesium, etc.).

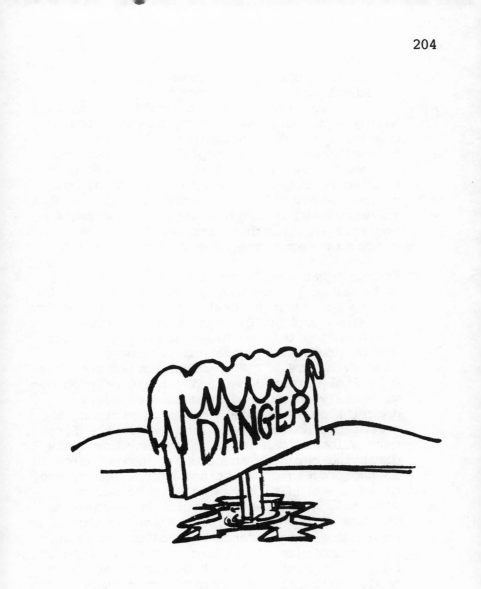

When in doubt, see the doctor.

Q. Should I go off vitamins when I do
    macrobiotics?
A. This is individual and you should discuss it
    with the doctor. Basically, macrobiotics
    does not recommend vitamin supplements.
    However, many of the people that we see are
    extremely low in certain nutrients. We have
    watched macrobiotics correct nutrients, but
    it has taken, oftentimes, six to twelve months
    to do so, and it might be better to correct
    yourself in a month or two and then
    discontinue so that you have a "head start".

    Don't forget that macrobiotics is a very
    old healing philosophy, and it is learning to
    modify and adapt to newly created 20th century
    diseases, such as E.I. and the multiple
    deficiencies that we have caused through our
    way of processing foods and our changes in
    dietary habits. The chemical environment has
    definitely created new and unheard of problems
    with newly formulated chemicals of every
    description in people's bodies disturbing the
    normal biochemical function. We're the first
    generation of mankind with so many chemicals
    deranging our body functions. Macrobiotics is
    in the process of adapting. For example, many
    of us are exquisitely sensitive to natural
    gas, and, of course, macrobiotics recommends
    the use of natural gas over electrical cooking
    because of interference with electro-magnetic
    fields and vital life force energy in foods.
    Many of us must cook with electric (and have
    healed with it). For many I would never
    recommend returning to gas.

Q. Should I go off my injections when I'm on
    macrobiotics?
A. Again, macrobiotics would say go off them as
    soon as you can, however, we have a
    specifically weak population that is

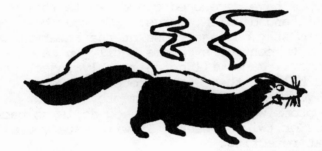

When you are discharging you will, from time to time, emit horrid odors. You might as well prepare your friends. I thought maybe they wouldn't notice. I was wrong.

genetically susceptible to developing chemical hypersensitivity. Furthermore hidden nutritional deficiencies can promote the spreading phenomenon leading to further sensitivities to foods, molds, Candida, and other chemicals.

Many needed injections for quite awhile in order to keep the total load sufficiently low enough to be able to cope. Some of us need them indefinitely. Remember not everyone may do their program as perfectly as they need to for their condition. And macrobiotics isn't some magic cure-all. People have developed cancer while they were on it and died (K. Burns). So your best bet is to stay on injections at the interval you need to control symptoms until you see the doctor. Many will go on monthly injections and hold it there for a couple of years. Then if you decide to abandon macro, or your symptoms worsen, all you need do is go back to once or twice a week. It will save you all that retesting.

Q. What if my chemical sensitivities get worse on macrobiotics?

A. That would be quite possible, and we have seen this in environmental medicine with a mere diet change. Sometimes it's a loss of adaptive enzymes or an unmasking that causes this. The problem is in deciding whether it's an actual discharge reaction or a real worsening of chemical sensitivity. You should see the doctor when this happens. It will help us learn about your individual system and whether your liver is really discharging. We may even be able to measure some old chemicals (pesticides, drugs, formaldehyde, etc.) as they come out of the fat storage into the blood on their way to the liver.

Q. How can I tell if I'm having a discharge
   reaction or symptoms?
A. The best way is to see the doctor and/or have
   some blood work done, but also bear in mind
   that when one is having a discharge, there
   is a certain mental set where even though
   you're having symptoms you have mental
   clarity which normally you would not have
   during these symptoms. You also have an
   unprecedented feeling of well-being or peace
   that you normally would not have with these
   types of symptoms.

Q. What if I need to take medication?
A. Macrobiotics attempts to detoxify the system
   and get rid of chemicals, just as we also try
   to keep people free of medication in
   environmental medicine. If you must take
   medication, however, do so; especially if you
   are a severe asthmatic. Never hesitate to
   take your medication if you feel you need it.
   Varying amounts of time are needed for people
   to heal sufficiently without their
   medications. Never risk making yourself
   dangerously sick. And when in doubt see the
   doctor.

Q. What if I need to stop my macrobiotic program?
A. Once you have started you should decide on a
   commitment for a specified period of time.
   Usually six months. If you stop and start,
   you may make yourself worse, and at best you
   will slow the healing process so much that
   you'll become disenchanted with the whole
   program and discontinue it. When in doubt,
   if you get caught in a bad situation, in a
   restaurant, order only steamed vegetables or
   mineral water or just don't eat.

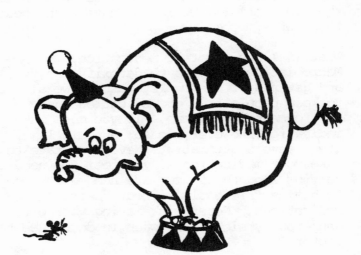

     Weight loss is effortless with macrobiotics.
If you are normal or underweight to begin with, you
will need closer supervision.

Q. What if I lose too much weight with
    macrobiotics?
A. Weight loss is to be expected, and you will
    lose in the first few months, and should.
    People will be telling you that you look awful
    and you should eat more. But just remind them
    that you're getting rid of old fat and
    chemicals, and then you're going to put back
    your fat again but with clean, organic foods
    and you will only be putting back as much fat
    as you actually need. If you find you have
    too much weight loss and cannot control it,
    you should see the doctor. Another clue that
    the weight loss is not detrimental is if you
    are feeling great.

Q. What evidence is there for macrobiotics?
A. There are a few papers on macrobiotics.
    The reference which has the most number in it
    is Michio Kushi's The Book of Macrobiotics
    (1987).

Q. Will I need my Nystatin and Vital Dophilus
    to treat my Candida on macrobiotics?
A. Remember, Candida is merely a symptom that
    you're not biochemically balanced. There is
    still a stressor present and you are not
    playing with a full deck. Once you have a
    healthier body, you'll be able to go off the
    Candida program and not have the symptoms.
    For example, you can take an antibiotic and
    not get Candida once you are healthy. Many
    people do. Also remember that a vast majority
    of the people with Candida are better right
    away, just off sugar. They have quickly
    relaxed their buffering system and removed one
    of the major drains on the system. Remember,
    too, meat keeps the sweet cravings alive.

Q.   Should I rotate on macrobiotics?
A.   Yes, you should, but in the beginning you'll
     be lucky to just do macrobiotics, much less
     rotate it. However, after about the sixth
     month, you'll probably be infinitely more
     sophisticated and able to rotate. I suspect
     we all should do that and macrobiotics does
     stress a varied diet. Remember, we still
     are part of the 21st century where we are
     capable of becoming sensitized to foods that
     we eat repeatedly. Ours is a genetically
     weaker and chemically more stressed breed of
     people than has ever been studied before.

Q.   What if macrobiotics isn't working?
A.   You should see the doctor and make sure you're
     doing things correctly. Some people do better
     with a tailor made program that is not in the
     50:25:10 percent ratio for G, G and B.

Q.   What if I don't tolerate any grains?
A.   This often happens with people with severe
     E.I. You may need to start with non-grain
     carbohydrates such as quinoa, amaranth,
     tapioca or buckwheat. Also, you may want to
     fast for three or four days and then try oats,
     barley, organic brown rice, or millet and see
     if you tolerate those once you are unloaded.
     If not, you'll need to go to the greens,
     squashes, and beans for starters. You'll most
     likely benefit from counseling help.

     One universal reactor was bedridden with pain
     and exhaustion when she was referred by the
     medical center. On the E.I. program she made
     remarkable improvement in her previously
     severe chemical sensitivity and Candida
     problems. She was out of bed, caring for the
     family and household. But just the smell of
     fabric softener sheets from neighbors' clothes
     dryers as she walked her children could
     trigger symptoms. She decided to go the next

step and eat macrobiotically. But she
developed severe exhaustion as though there
were some severe deficiency. However, she
found the solution in eating broken grains.
In other words, by grinding the grains into
flours and making pancakes, she began deriving
relief from more E.I. symptoms and without the
weakness. Clearly she has a digestive
problem, possibly resistant Candida, like the
dreaded C. tropicalis (see The E.I.
Syndrome for explanation).

Q. How important is it to phase out my injections
under medical supervision?
A. Very. It may be the difference between
struggling through a tough discharge of weeks
or months, or sailing through a mild one.
Most of us who work cannot afford to take off
several weeks to be ill.

First, remember that some people we have seen
could not even begin to clear in the first
place on macrobiotics without reducing their
total load (see The E.I. Syndrome for
explanation). This total load includes
chemically less-contaminated food and air. It
also includes pushing the body to make
blocking antibodies and T suppressor cells to
turn off an abnormal reactivity to air borne
molds. Many people were less sensitive to
foods, Candida or chemicals just as soon as
they began unloading with titrated injections
to the newer molds.

Secondly, there is the question of immunologic
memory. When someone gets measles or the
immunization, they usually have lifelong
immunity to it. The body remembers to produce
those antibodies for years to come. The
immunologic memory is good. With tetanus,
flus and other immune stimulators there is

varying individual response. Some people
remember to make antibodies for years, others
only a few months.

Remember, a carefully titrated allergy
injection contains nothing more that what you
would normally breath anyway: it's just in a
route and dose that stimulates your body to
produce the helpful or blocking antibody (IgG)
as opposed to the harmful one (IgE). In
general, each person is highly individual and
should assess this with the doctor to minimize
you having to retest at some time.

Some people will require a periodic reminder
to boost the immune system, others will not.
As long as it's there to keep the body
unloaded enough to get on with the work of
healing, that is all that matters.

Q.   What about some of the herb baths that are
     recommended?
A.   Again we must balance 20th century "faux pas"
     against benefit. Most municipal U.S. waters
     contain levels of chlorine that make many
     people with E.I. ill. To deliberately immerse
     your body in it if you know you react, is
     silly. There are a couple hundred other
     chemicals in it as well. Chloroform and
     trichloroethylene can be volatilized just from
     the shower spray. You will need to assess
     your severity of sensitivity and the degree of
     contamination of your water to decide if the
     benefits or the baths outweigh the risk.

Q.   What if I don't tolerate any foods?
A.   You may need to start on food injections and
     a rare food rotated diet in order to be able
     to tolerate foods, then you can gradually
     swing into a more macrobiotic routine. Go
     back and assess your total load and follow the
     E.I. checklist. If you're too chemically
     overloaded you'll never tolerate foods.

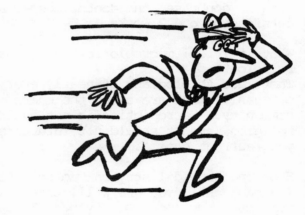

    Diarrhea is a common discharge symptom. When
in doubt, see the doctor.

Q. What if I get worse while I'm on macrobiotics?
    What if I get very ill, have excessive weight
    loss, feel awful and have constant symptoms?
A. Then you should see the doctor so that it can
    be determined why you are worse. You should
    also check that you are chewing your
    foods well, that you have the correct
    proportions, and that you are not overeating.
    Also, be sure that your foods are mostly
    organic, and if you are still having
    trouble, you should definitely see the doctor.

Q. What if I am having chronic diarrhea?
A. When in doubt see the doctor, especially if it
    persists beyond 2 weeks.

Q. What if I feel macrobiotics is against my
    religion?
A. There are theologians of nearly every
    persuasion that are among the macrobiotic
    community. Macrobiotics is not against any
    religion, and it should not interfere with
    your current choice.

Q. How long should I stay on macrobiotics?
A. At least until you are well, then I would be
    very cautious about modifying. I would
    suggest you read Colbin's, Food and Healing,
    and try to modify in terms of this, rather
    than returning to your canned fare. Hopefully
    you will have learned so much about yourself
    that you will not really abandon but merely
    modify.

    Remember some people get dramatically worse
    once they veer from this program. This is
    partly because of loss of adaptation. A first
    cigarette makes one ill, the second is better,
    and the rest is ancient history. Actually it
    is wonderful that you feel sick in a newly
    painted room. Who wants a blood stream with

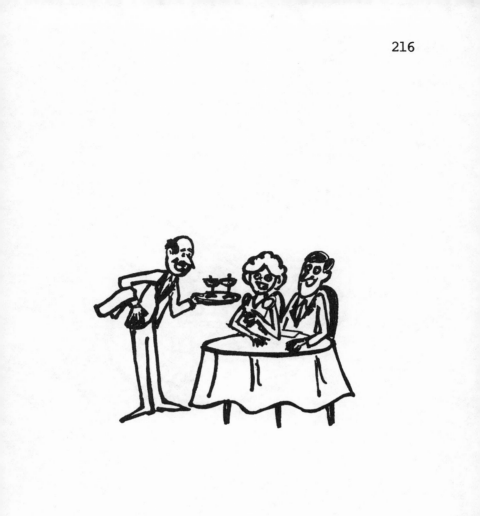

As long as you pay attention to your stage of treatment, you can go anywhere. You just need to realize what you can and can't have. Then it's simple. You know right away if you should bring your own food or not. Remember you're going for the social fun, not the actual food.

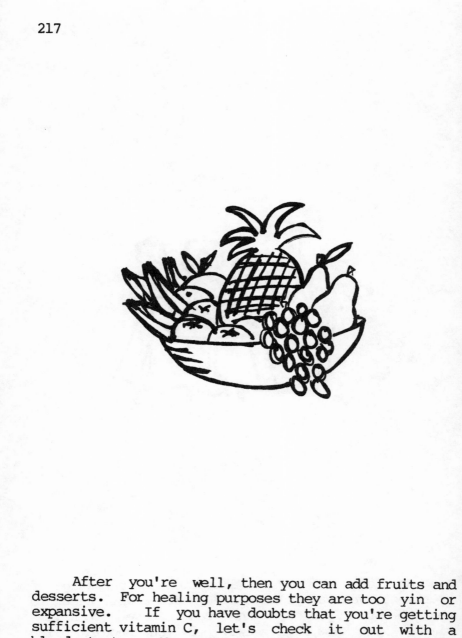

After you're well, then you can add fruits and desserts. For healing purposes they are too yin or expansive. If you have doubts that you're getting sufficient vitamin C, let's check it out with a blood test. My motto: When in doubt, check it out.

carcinogenic volatile organic hydrocarbons in it? Just because others may have adaptive enzymes that allow them to tolerate such exposures doesn't make them any less resistant to the potential long term effects.

Q. What if I hate the food?
A. If you don't feel peaceful and serene on the program, I would suggest that you visit the East West Center and have some of their meals. Or have meals prepared by the members who cook well macrobiotically, and determine if it's your neophyte cooking that is uninspiring. There are several good macro cooks who will cater; try them out. Also be sure to check your proportions or balance. And then again, remember that macrobiotics is not for everyone; nothing is.

Q. What do I do when I want to go somewhere?
A. You must plan since the average American cuisine is not healthfully oriented. I usually have some umeboshi-nori rolls or boiled peeled almonds or roasted pumpkin seeds ready so that I could dash off for several hours, and if I ended up in a restaurant I would have something to nibble on.

Q. Why don't I just go vegetarian?
A. There are many vegetarians who are extremely unhealthy. Many of them are overtly obese. Some of them are very vitamin depleted. This is because many of them are not knowledgeable about good nutrition and under the guise of not eating meat, they eat a tremendous amount of wheat products often flavored with honey. However, on an airplane or in some restaurants, vegetarian would provide a partial substitute for you and be far better than all of the dairy, meats, and processed foods that you would get in the normal restaurant fare.

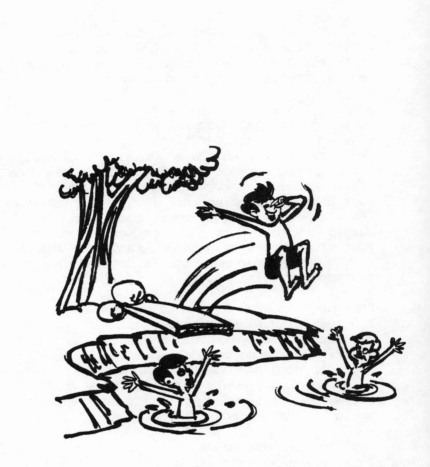

Exercise is important:

(1) it helps detoxify
(2) it helps stave off depression
(3) it improves body tone
(4) it adds to your confidence and concentration

Q. What if I modify the macrobiotics?
A. In the first three to six months I would not modify anything, because you are trying to see how much of your symptoms you can simmer down with a program that has taken years to work out.

Q. Why are there no famous octogenarian macrobiotic people?
A. This question bothered me, as well, for I know many leaders in the field of clinical ecology who are in their 80's and appear healthier than many people in their 60's. But I have not seen this in macrobiotics and it disturbs me. I hope we will have an answer soon. Lima Ohsawa (wife of Georges)is 90 and in admirable condition. He, however, died before 70.

Q. What do I do if I feel my program doesn't have much supervision?
A. You should see the doctor so that the details of your program and your questions can be dealt with more fully.

Q. How do I make my journey to wellness go faster?
A. Many things will slow you up. Probably the best things to speed you up will be to eat less and lose more weight and generally eat 50 to 60 percent rice. Moderate exercise, sweating, massage, ginger compresses, meditation and other adjuncts also aid to speed things up. And, of course, keep your life ecologically clean. If you are overburdened by a chemically contaminated environment you may forever retard healing.

Q. How do I know if I'm doing things correctly? Does anyone make house calls?
A. At this point we don't have anyone that does. Your best bet would be to write out your menu

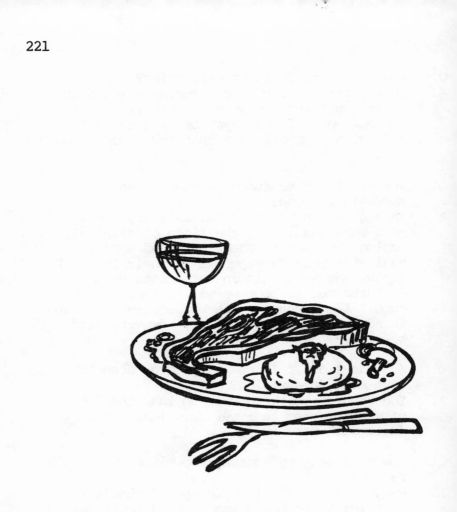

Some people need meat. Some people don't. It's very simple, if you just listen to your body. But you'll grossly distort its signaling system by feeding it plastic food.

and proportions of foods that are ingested for each meal and then share that with your counselor or the doctor.

Q. Could I die from macrobiotics?
A. I have never heard of this happening on the diet outlined in here, but if at anytime you just plain don't feel well you should see the doctor. An examination plus specific mineral, vitamin, organ enzyme and other blood tests can be checked. Perhaps you have a deficiency that's been unrecognized in the past. If anything should kill you, it's what you have eaten in the past! And, there is always a possibility of developing a new condition for which modern acute care medicine is suited.

Years ago some people died who stupidly ate only brown rice. That scenario has become a legend among people who malign macrobiotics without fully understanding it.

Q. Could I get deficient on macrobiotics?
A. Yes, but macrobiotics stresses variety, just as we in environmental medicine stress rotation. It gives you much more variety and less chance of developing deficiencies than does the S.A.D. (Standard American Diet). When in doubt, we should check your levels. Good indicators of your status would be a vitamin A, B12, B1, C, an rbc zinc, rbc magnesium, copper and selenium for starters.

Q. When do I branch out?
A. After you have gone through a couple of discharges and you have vastly improved some of your major symptoms, then you can start eating a more lenient diet.

Q. When do I have my first steak?
A. Possibly in a year, possibly never. It depends very much on the person and his needs.

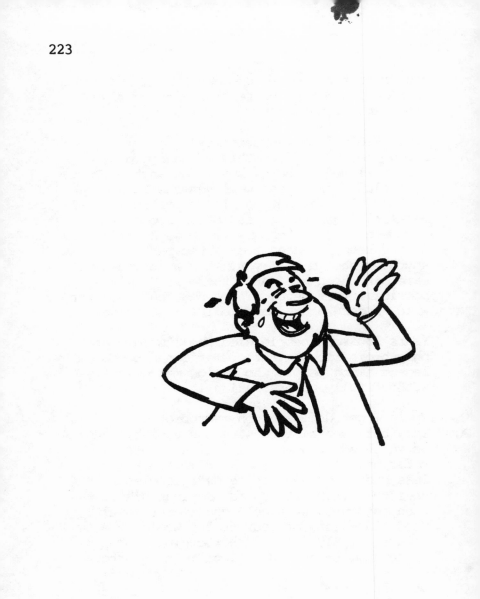

A buddy is indispensable. It's much more fun to have someone to laugh with. And as you both devour the more advanced macro books, you'll teach one another.

Hopefully, with your macrobiotic reading and experimentation with the diet, you will see that you feel better than you have ever in your life, and it will change you so that you will never be the same again. The same thing happens with people who go through the rare food, rotation diet to identify food allergies and learn about processed foods and nutrient deficiencies. Even though they may not stay on a rare food, rotated diet all of their lives, or they may not stay on a Candida diet all of their lives, they have learned so much that they could never go back to the junk food life that they had had in the past. They are forever changed or altered for the good. When you are healed, you will have steaks and assess how you feel. You will be able to listen to your body and determine if you need meat or not. Some people must have it. Either they do heavy work, or work in the cold, or get so bland on greens that they bore themselves.

Q. What do I do if I am fantasizing about ice cream?
A. Anne Marie Colbin's book, <u>Food</u> <u>and</u> <u>Healing</u>, has many suggestions for cravings; umeboshi (plums), "rice cream", and better balancing of your diet are some of the many things that can be done when you have cravings. Remember a craving is a good thing, because it is a clue that you are out of balance. It is a warning before illness and degenerative problems occur.

Q. Do I need a buddy?
A. Absolutely. This makes everything in life easier. If you can find someone who is going to go on the program with you, that you can confer with each day, that you can share expenses with when you buy bulk at a co-op, that you split up shopping with for strange

items, it always makes things easier. Also,
it's always nice to have someone that you can
laugh with.

Q. How long should I let bad symptoms go on?
A. No more than two weeks if it's a bad symptom
such as chronic coughing or congestion, or
achiness, or diarrhea. If something like
asthma or diarrhea is very bad, you may only
be able to let it go a day or two, then you
should be checked to determine if it's a
discharge phenomenon or not.

Q. Why don't I just stay on the same diet that
made me well?
A. Because the pendulum will always swing to
the opposite side sooner or later and then
you'll feel lousy because of what you're
eating. In other words, take people who have
Candida. They feel wonderful in the first
few weeks or months when they get off so many
sweets. Then the pendulum swings to the
opposite end where they are having a
proportionately larger amount of meats and
they begin to feel lousy because of this.
There is no diet that is great for everyone,
and likewise even when a person finds a diet
that is great for him, it does
not mean that it will remain great for him.
Through all levels of stress and environmental
conditions, his needs change, his seasons
change, his body changes. The diet that makes
you well, is not necessarily the one that you
should stay on. Besides the diet that makes
you well is usually quite restricted, and the
diet you want for maintenance is infinitely
more varied and lenient.

Remember when we correct vitamin deficiencies,
we first put people on a corrective supplement
program which is extremely unbalanced, but it
must be unbalanced to balance the extreme

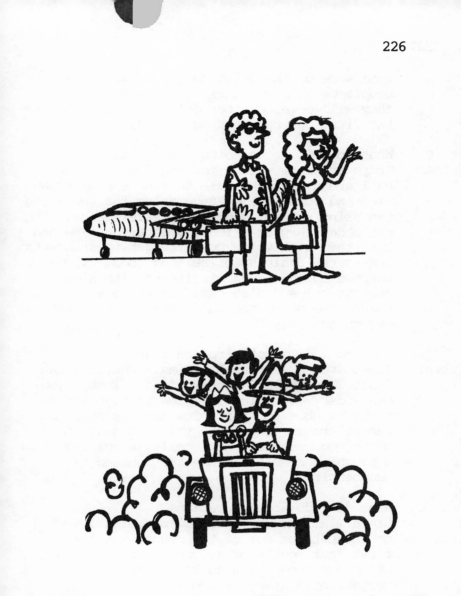

Vacations, large or small, just take more planning. There are publications in <u>Macromuse</u> magazine you can order that give locations of vegetarian/macrobiotic restaurants and services all over the world. You could always bring brown rice and have your hotel cook it for you (or bring a hot plate and cook your own when you need balance).

imbalance of the deficiency. If we leave people on this corrective program, however, they will develop other deficiencies once the first one has been corrected.

Q. What do I do about going out to dinner?
A. There are many things you can do. You can call ahead and make sure they have some brown rice and some steamed vegetables for you. You can bring some of your own little snacks. You can order them at a local vegetarian cafe and take them with you. Don't forget, restaurants are in the business of selling food. They adapted to the needs of clients with high cholesterol and diabetes. If there's a need, they'll adapt to the call from those eating macrobiotically.

Q. What do I do about airplane travel?
A. There are three possibilities. One, you can fast. Two, bring your own food. Three, you can order vegetarian and pick through and maybe be able to find a few nibbles that you can tolerate. Your best thing is just to bring your umeboshi-nori rolls, since the umeboshi can help balance the inhaled xenobiotics.

Q. What do I do about vacations?
A. Since I am the universal guinea pig, I went on three trips out of the country in the first four months of my program and took all of my own food. I also took some to restaurants; it can be done.

Q. What happens if I eat meat or fruit or sweets, bread, or ice cream?
A. There are a number of things that can happen. One, you can slow up your program. Two, you can create an imbalance that will then trigger other cravings. Three, you can set your

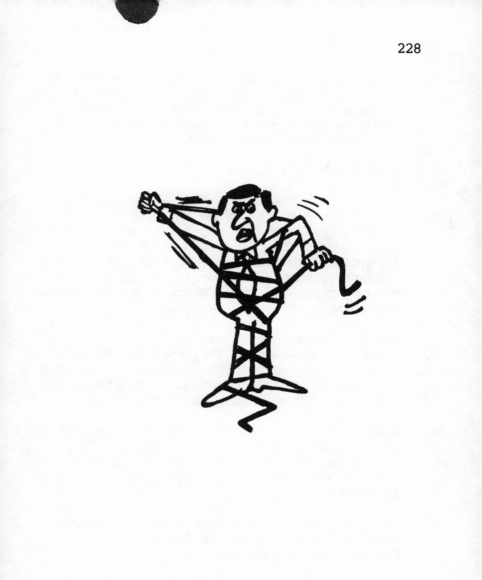

If you're not happy on macrobiotics, you'd better see your counselor or the doctor. You may be eating wrong.

progress back for weeks. Four, it means you missed a marvelous opportunity to learn how to correct an imbalance that you had, since an uncontrollable craving means there is an imbalance that needs correcting.

Q. Should I keep a diary?
A. Yes.

Q. Should I put my family on the diet?
A. It all depends on how eager they are to do it. I would not force it on anybody. Oftentimes, you can ease the foods into the meal plan and frequently people will become interested when they see your wellness materialize.

Q. How do I know I've detoxed?
A. You'll know because you'll feel better and better after each discharge reaction and have progressively fewer symptoms to endure as you tolerate a broader range of exposures.

Q. What if I get severely depressed or irritable?
A. This may be a symptom or a discharge and you should see the doctor when you're in doubt since blood tests can be done to discern which is present.

Q. What do I do if I get severe pain or severe weakness or severe weight loss?
A. See the doctor when in doubt.

Q. Why are the men in macrobiotics so skinny? No wonder they're all pacifists. I need a diet to suit my build.
A. There are robust macro men, but yes many are slight of build, and I don't have an answer. I suspect the answer lies somewhere in the fact that oriental men do not possess the same body habitus as, for example, a German or Swede.

As you will see, you can eat far more inexpensively with macro as compared with the Standard American fare or rare food organic rotation.

Therefore, modification of the diet may be in order for some nationalities.

It's ironic that Ohsawa lectured in France on macrobiotics telling them to eat by the laws of nature and the foods that were indigenous to the area. No wonder many ignored him. How much daikon, wakame, rice, and miso are indigenous to France? There are apparent incongruities. All I know is there is a system here that works well for healing, and that it can and must eventually be modified for use by greater numbers.

Q. Are macrobiotic foods irradiated?
A. That's a tough question. Proponents of food irradiation try to get as little labeling as possible and increasingly more items are being OK'd for irradiation. As you know, the process destroys a significant portion of vitamins and creates new untested chemicals called "unique radiolytic products" (U.R.P.).

Q. Is mercury toxicity a problem with the seaweeds?
A. I don't know, but it's one of the minerals we'll be investigating as we assess people eating macrobiotically.

Q. What if I'm constipated?
A. Constipation on macrobiotics suggests the need for a colonoscopy and bowel X-ray series, for correction of constipation is usually one of the first benefits. Movements become regular, simple, painless, and odorless; most Americans could evacuate the house with the odor of their bowel movements. Constipation suggests putrefaction in the gut. Toxins will be absorbed into the blood stream. If your bowel movements are not daily, soft, sweet smelling or odorless, (unless discharging), you should see the doctor.

Q.   Can I use tap water in my cooking?
A.   No. Most U.S. municipalities have way too
     many chemicals in their water nowadays. The
     chlorine level some mornings at my home in the
     tap water at my home smells like pure Clorox
     (R) some mornings. The analysis of
     xenobiotics for many cities across the U.S.
     reveals about 500 chemicals. Some are
     intentionally added to mask others that are
     expensive or impossible to get rid of.
     Industrial contamination of water tables is
     rampant in the U.S. Many of the chemicals are
     hydrocarbons which, of course, are free
     radical sources. In other words, they create
     crazy naked electrons in the body which charge
     around aimlessly leaving destruction in their
     pathways. The membrane and protein
     destruction that results can potentiate aging,
     allergies, degenerative diseases, mutation and
     cancer (see The E.I. Syndrome).

Q.   I hesitate to ask but, how do you
     cook brown rice?
A.   Most of us did not know. There are many fine
     cookbooks and courses, but to speed up your
     initiation: Wash 2 cups brown rice in a
     colander, sort for stones, put in pressure
     cooker. Add 3 cups clean water, a pinch of
     salt, and turn on high. In about 5-10 minutes
     the whistle will blow. Put heat dissipater
     between cooker and burner and turn to lowest
     setting for 40 minutes. When timer goes off,
     remove from burner, prop fork under vent to
     let off steam. Voila!

Q.   I've eaten according to Macro rules and I
     don't see any difference?
A.   No one therapy in the world is for everyone.
     But the commonest reasons for failure are not
     watching the proportions, having poor
     environmental controls (see the E.I.
     Syndrome), and failure to reduce stress. The

latter should include an enjoyable exercise program, meditation, reflective lifestyle modifications, a spiritual reassessment and self-nurturing. You must start doing loving things for yourself and others each day.

Do a periodic attitudinal assessment. See food as a friend, as a positive healing tool, not as an enemy and something that will bring on reactions. Find out what's really bugging you in life and get rid of it. Many people harbor subconscious insecurities, anger (which fosters guilt) and hurt which keeps "eating at" them. These demons must be devoured so you're once more as mentally free as a child. Only then can your playful, creative, and loving instincts emerge.

Rx: Bring laughter into yours and someone else's life every day.

Q. Now that you are into health, does this mean you trade your high heels and suits in for construction boots and long skirts?
A. There's much to be said for a back to nature lifestyle, stress reduction, non-conformity, lessened obsession with obtaining all the accoutrements of suburban society. But on the flip side, we owe the movers and shakers more than we could ever hope to repay. I hope health will become so "in", that a 3-piece suit does not look out of place in stores where sacks of grains and beans predominate.

Q. How about a quick synopsis?
A. Cut out meats and sweets.
Substitute grains and greens.
Work into grains, greens and beans, seeds and (sea)weeds, roots and "fruits". Don't forget miso soup once or twice a day once you begin to tolerate it.
Chew each mouthful well.

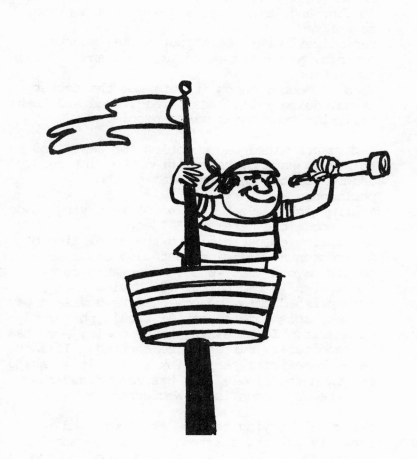

Keep a look out for bum excuses. If you don't have time for macro, maybe you just plain don't choose to make time for wellness at this point in life under any conditions. You're just not sick enough.

Watch your proportions: 50-25-10% of G, G,
and B, or 50:50 of grains:vegetables.
Check your nutritional levels.
Periodically evaluate your progress with the
doctor, and learn what's new on the horizon,
as well.
Periodically re-assess your goals, short-
comings, accomplishments, methods and
motivation.
When in doubt, check it out; see the doctor
if not doing well. Read, read, read and then
talk with successful macro people.

Q. I have practiced macrobiotics for years and
think you have oversimplified the diet and
underestimated the remainder of the
philosophy.

A. You're right. Bear in mind we're trying to do
the impossible here: (1) Identify a
discipline compatible with the discipline of
environmental medicine that also can take
people beyond what we have been able to
accomplish in the past. (2) Having
accomplished this, we now need to devise a way
to make this foreign and difficult philosophy
palatable. In attaining these goals, much has
to temporarily suffer or be shorted. If macro
is as beneficial as I think it is, it's taking
off much too slowly. It has many drawbacks
for the yet unconvinced Westerner.

I'm merely trying to show the logic and
simplify getting started. If the person
starts to get the results he's been looking
for, he'll be hooked and go for perfection,
learning all he can. Any one who gets that
far has to realize he carries the ball and we
cannot spoon-feed him the rest of the way. We
can match him with the most suitable
counselor,we can help him monitor and modify,
but he does the work and must also be
constantly learning. MB broadens a person's

awareness and urges him to explore other alternative therapies if macro does not suit him.

Q. I found the diet to be the least helpful and the philosophy to be my mainstay.
A. True. For some, there is even progressive emotional discharge as they relive aspects of the past.

Q. Isn't it true that one has to embrace totally the philosophy of macrobiotics to get well?
A. There is wide biochemical variability. Some people need meat. There is a wide range of sickness. Many get better with diet alone. That's probably due to the fact that it's the perfect rare food diet and for the most part avoids the extremes of acid/alkaline, and avoids processed foods, concentrating on whole, vital foods. Clearly, the philosophical attitude of macrobiotics provides even further benefit. There is never a reason for anger, jealousy, depression, or self-pity when you believe (1) nothing is totally yang (there is some good in everything), (2) sickness is a good thing; it's the body's way of balancing or discharging, and (3) you are responsible for your illnesses, but on the other hand you have the power to heal them. As well, there are many additional benefits that extend to the cosmic man. And of course on the other end of the spectrum are many other pluses; seeing food as friend, not as an enemy, living closer to nature so that awareness and appreciation blossom, etc.

Q. I've heard macrobiotics is very strict.
A. I've heard Mr. Kushi teaching a class to aspiring counselors in healing. On one hand, he insists that MB is not rigid, but the broadest, most flexible diet there is, that

there are no forbidden foods. And indeed, a
wide variety is recommended. On the other
hand, he tells them if they eat chicken or
meat, or eat "chaotically", such as while
working at one's desk, this reflects a shallow
life and indicates they are not suitable to be
counselors.

Many aspects of the philosophy are right in
line with the positivity and creative
visualization techniques that the field of
psychoneuoimmunology would suggest. Symptoms
are viewed without paralyzing fear: a cancer
is seen as a localization of harmful cells so
they can be gotten rid of. All sickness
benefits men, for the mechanism of symptoms is
to make the patient better. He must have
faith in this constant struggle for harmony
with nature. We should be grateful for
symptoms, or we would have become extinct
long ago if we hadn't had a way of discharging
our excesses. It is because of sickness that
mankind survives. When sickness is seen as
bad, he continues, there is no gratitude, no
self-reflection to see how you can make
yourself better. Macrobiotics fosters
tolerance, a spirituality if you will.

But this is carried even further where they
are anti-immunization, (fine if the whole
world is macrobiotic, but if one person is
not, he'll start an epidemic, theoretically),
no medical system, no military weapons (they
feel aggression comes from eating meat), etc.
There are many arguments that corporate
America could counter with. I'm not certain
if one needs to be a pacifist in order to
fulfill the macrobiotic ideal. You can decide
how much of the philosophy suits you. The
peace of mind and faith seem to suit many.

Q. This is ridiculous, how could one possibly
    hope to heal, for example, a coronary artery
    plugged by arteriosclerosis?
A. The medical profession has trained us as
    physicians to perform more like auto
    mechanics. We see a malfunction and replace
    the part. It's easier often than restoring
    the old. The problem is, your body is not a
    car.

Our mechanical view is pervasive----if one has
a case of bad colitis, cut out the bowel and
throw it away (it's practically heresy to look
for a hidden food allergy). You have fluids
in the ear canals? Puncture the tympanic
membrane and put in a drain tube.

With coronary artery disease the same
mechanical view is held when drugs fail. Cut
out the arteries and put in some from the leg
or just ream out the old ones. A recent
publication (Hospital Practice, May 15,
1988) by a Mayo Clinic researcher shows there
are receptors in those blood vessels that
cause relaxation of the vessel when the lining
is healed. These very same receptors cause
contraction when the vessel wall is inflamed.
But what simmers down inflammation more
definitively than a search for ecologic
triggers and a good healing diet?
Furthermore, studies show that there is less
reactivity and inflammation of vessels seen
with Max EPA (eicosopentaenoic acid, see The
E.I. Syndrome) than with aspirin. But this
information takes time to reach those
cardiologists who are not yet even advocating
avoiding all processed foods that contain
hydrogenated vegetable oil. Some of this oil
contains coconut oil which is 88% saturated
fat (beef is only 40%, egg 33%). It's ironic

that the "low cholesterol" plastic foods, like
artificial coffee creamers, are actually
recommended by hospital dieticians for
patients with dangerously compromised coronary
arteries.

Q. How can something you eat affect your moods?
A. There are many levels on which this occurs.
First is by a direct allergy, second is by
affecting balance and pH, and third by having
disharmonious electromagnetic frequencies
(phenolics). Also there are receptors for
many intestinal messengers, like vasoactive
intestinal peptide in the gut, lung and brain
for example. All the data is not in, but
clearly reactions in the gut are transmitted
to brain receptors. Lastly there is the
psychogenic taste gratification aspect.

Q. Can zinc deficiency cause AIDS?
A. It is interesting that most AIDS victims in
whom an rbc zinc is tested are deficient.
Zinc is crucial for synthesis of a thymic
factor whose deficiency does cause AIDS. It
certainly could be one of the vulnerability
factors that set the stage.

Q. As a physician who studied over 9 years, and
practiced over 18 years, how can you recommend
something where lay counselors diagnose such
idiotic things as mineral deficiencies without
so much as a blood test?
A. Much of it I agree, does sound bizarre by our
standards, but when you observe people, for
example, having elevated liver enzymes when
they are supposedly going through a liver
discharge, it's mighty convincing. Much is
common sense, however. For example they look
at fingernails for splitting and breaking,
hair for dryness, frizziness and breaking and
suspect mineral deficiencies. They add more
seaweeds and the nails and hair change in 6
months. Doctors could do this as well,

especially since they have all the tests of
proof available to them.

I have witnessed a skilled counselor diagnose
liver problem in a nurse with normal liver
chemistries. The diagnosis was made by noting
the faintest yellowness in the medial sclera
(whites of the eyes on the nose side). And
the counselor was correct since the nurse had
just gotten over a severe case of shingles
that had caused severe pain in that area.

What gets me is how was all this was figured
out years ago. They go further and attribute
specific emotions to specific organs: anger
for the liver, fear for the kidney. And darn
if it doesn't pan out much of the time. When
patients are no longer as chemically reactive
or up urinating all night, those emotions
mellow out. I have felt it in myself and
observed it in others as well.

Fascinating as it is, I can't agree with all
of it yet. I see myself as a negotiator,
merely attempting to get West to look at East.
There's no question the West's strength is
acute care medicine and the East's is chronic
disease. Why can't we enjoy the best of each?

Q.   My counselor insists I use miso, but it makes
     my Candida symptoms worse.
A.   It should and you need to have a more up to
     date counselor selected for you. Mr. Kushi in
     his book, Allergies, shows the best
     understanding of environmental illness I have
     ever seen by a non-ecologist. So perhaps your
     counselor has not studied long enough, and for
     sure, hasn't had too much experience with E.I.
     or Candida.

     When you're well, you'll have no problem
     listening to your body. You may feel

exhausted for example, at a change of season,
and find you get a boost from some fish or
chicken. You can eventually learn how
to eat to feel great all the time. Don't
forget you're in a constant state of flux, as
are the seasons and your environment. This
requires monitoring and modification.

Q. I've heard of people getting cancer while on
    macrobiotics.
A. In this decade, one of the staff (Ken Burns)
    of MACROMUSE (a macrobiotic magazine), was
    under 50, acquired and died of cancer, and he
    had been macrobiotic for many years prior to
    this. On the other hand, Dirk Benedict, a
    handsome T.V. actor developed his cancer while
    on macro and cured his cancer while on
    macrobiotics (The Kamikazi Cowboy is his
    story). These types of questions I do not
    have an answer for. Then there's another
    book about a person who had cancer of the
    pancreas. He cleared on macrobiotics,
    but he later died of pneumonia. On autopsy
    they were delighted to report that he died of
    pneumonia and that the pancreas was totally
    free of cancer. Again, I'm perplexed why the
    person died of pneumonia. Why couldn't a
    simple pneumonia be conquered if progress was
    so good with macrobiotics that the pancreatic
    cancer was cleared? Granted, everyone has to
    die sometime.

Q. How much should I eat?
A. You should only eat to about 80 percent of
    your satiety, especially if you are
    overweight. The less you eat the quicker you
    will have a discharge because you will be
    getting rid of fats which contain many of the
    xenobiotics (foreign chemicals).

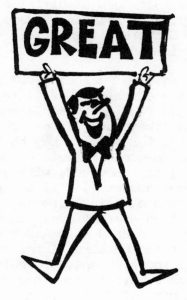

Regardless of whether you become a full-fledged macrobiotic convert or not, by learning about it and trying it, you have introduced yourself to a new level of wellness. I'll bet you include more whole grains, greens, and beans than you did prior. Even if it's only once or twice a week, it's better than none, which is what most of us had before. So you can't lose.

Q. How do you determine if I'm having a
    spontaneous depuration (detoxification or
    an actual discharge reaction) or symptoms?
A. Vitamin and mineral levels, enzyme levels of
    organs, including liver enzymes and a gamma
    glutamyl transaminase are some of the useful
    parameters that help us differentiate, and
    we're working on building a data base that
    will help doctors differentiate even more
    precisely in the future.

Q. What if I fail on macrobiotics?
A. There's no such thing as failure and you
    should avoid feeding yourself negative
    vibrations like that. If macrobiotics does
    not work out for you, it may be that you are a
    person who does not need it or chooses not to
    do the program. However, with all that you
    have learned and read, I'll bet that you
    have more whole grains, greens, and beans in
    your diet than ever before. In other words,
    once you have passed this way you are forever
    changed for the better. I for one rarely had
    any green, roots, beans, or whole grains.
    Even though I may not remain macro all my
    life, you can bet I'll have a healthy
    proportion of them forever. Most of us had
    a monotonous diet of bread, cheese, and wine,
    beef and sweets.

Q. What if there's no difference or no
    improvement after three months?
A. Then you should make sure that you have
    reduced your excess weight, watched your
    proportions and checked with the doctor.

Q. How do I know if I would benefit from
    macrobiotics?
A. You never really know until you try it, but
    most people are going through life at half
    mast because they don't really know what
    wellness feels like. It's much like a child

who is born with defective vision. He never
knows that the rest of the world sees a much
greater array than he does until someone fits
him with a pair of glasses. If you don't have
a great appetite for simple food, if you
can't fall asleep within five minutes, if you
don't have a good memory and a good sense of
humor, precision of thought and action,
creativity, enthusiasm and freedom of fatigue,
then you may find that through the macrobiotic
system of eating that you could feel a great
deal better. Also, if you need any more than
six hours of sleep a night, it's worthwhile to
evaluate the program.

Don't forget that conventional medicine only
recognizes endstage symptoms. It totally
ignores and even derides the notion that
early symptoms or subtle symptoms are of
any importance. However, every symptom is
a potential warning of more severe problems
to follow. Ask any heart attack victim.
Most of them just had a vague feeling of
unwellness and excessive tiredness the
week before they had their grand slam
heart attack. And, of course, for years prior
to this, they ate the wrong foods and many did
not enjoy a fully exuberant state of wellness.
If you can't awaken cheery, playful, and
laughing in the morning and truly say, "I feel
wonderful," then it behooves you to evaluate
the macrobiotic way.

Q. How did I get E.I.?
A. There are multiple factors at play in the
    development of E.I. One is heredity. Super-
    imposed on that usually is poor nutrition
    from years of eating processed foods or a lot
    of sweets. Then the detoxification system
    starts to peter out because of missing
    nutrients, such as zinc. Then the psychic
    stage may also be set with all of the mental

garbage that we carry around. Feelings of insecurity, guilt, jealousy, anger, are all very detrimental to the psychoneuroimmune system. Or there can be a tremendous emotional upset such as a divorce or a death, and of course there can be the monotonous diet of the same processed foods all the time, eventually triggering the upset of the apple cart. Candida sensitivity through many fermented and sweetened foods following antibiotics is a well known trigger. And, of course, many chemical hypersensitivities can start the landslide that we are all so familiar with; a new office, a new home, renovations, and the like.

Q. How long did it take me to get E.I.?
A. Probably, much like most other diseases, it is something that built up over the years, not something that came suddenly. The problem is that our sudden awareness of the disease only came about because of an eventual collapse of one of our body's systems. But the process had been building for years, just as it does in people with heart attacks, arteriosclerosis, diabetes, arthritis, colitis, cancer, etc.

We often speak of a heart attack as some disease that happened in five minutes. Quite the contrary, it had been building a long time. Likewise reversing the pathology should not consist solely of a quick fix with a pocketful of pills. Healing takes consistent intentional care over a long period of time.

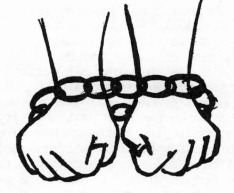

If your hands are tied and you become stuck at a stage with no progress, see the doctor. Keep good records of what you did that brought you to new levels of wellness. They will provide clues to your biochemistry.

Q. Why did I have to read all that nutritional detoxification biochemistry? It seems like there are two separate books here: one on nutrition and one on macrobiotics.

A. (1) We are the first (experimental) generation of people fed such devitalized foods and simultaneously exposed to so many chemicals. We break all the rules of medicine, and macrobiotics as well.

(2) As we realize that the responsibility for true health and healing lies with the individual, we have a further responsibility to educate.

(3) Because of these factors, plus tremendous individual biochemical variation and constant new research findings, it appears prudent for each person to understand the need for guidance in monitoring and modifying his program. The complexity becomes self-evident.

Q. Since I have E.I. am I more prone to cancer?

A. Usually people with E.I. are more prone to immune diseases such as arthritis, colitis, lupus, multiple sclerosis, and people with cancer and AIDS tend to be on the other end of the spectrum of immune dysfunction. Usually with cancer and AIDS the T helper cells are deficient. Deficient T helper cells is very serious and leaves one vulnerable to fatal illness when exposed to bacteria and fungi that don't normally affect people. For example, people with cancers and AIDS often die of Pneumocystis carinii pneumonia.

Normal healthy people and those with allergy, E.I., or autoimmune diseases are normally not affected by these organisms. However, their defect of poor T suppressor cells leads to the making of antibodies to just about everything in sight including their own tissues. In other words, the suppression or control of antibody response is lacking. Hence exaggerated response occurs to dusts, molds (Candida), pollens, foods and chemicals that normally would be harmless to others.

Q. Why is there such controversy in medicine regarding macrobiotics?

A. As with any therapy that takes control away from the doctor, and that most doctors are untrained in, and that does not make any money for drug companies, it does not receive any medical attention. Therefore, there's no research money. Therefore, there's no proof. Therefore, it is easily discredited.

Also, most acute care therapies are proven with double blind tests. This is easy if you're looking at the effect of one medicine. That means neither the doctor nor the patient knows if he is receiving the real medicine or nothing (a placebo or "sugar" pill). Only at the end of the study is the code broken. Hence double blind studies have become the gold standard. But that's a shortsighted view. How can you double blind the lifestyle and diet changes of E.I. and macrobiotics?

Q. Why are there so many alternatives to health?

A. You're right, there are many roads to "roam" (pardon the pun). I've seen people totally heal E.I. with macrobiotics, with prayer, with divorce, with nothing, with correcting their nutrient deficiencies, with injections to just foods, molds, or chemicals, correction of their Candida problem, and all of the above. I know of people who are trying to heal with the Gerson therapy, and I know of people who are much better having had polarity therapy, phenolics, and bioenergetic therapies.

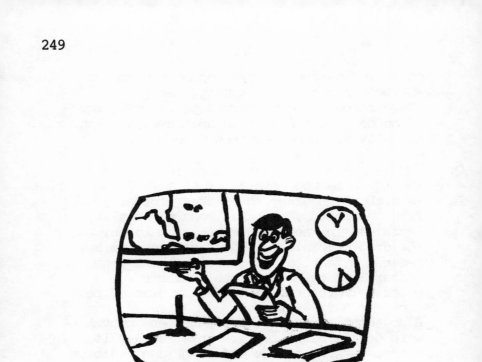

As you've learned through E.I., medical controversy is usually based on money and ego, not merely science.

We merely began by trying to find something that has a pretty good track record that also is more or less workable for the person with severe E.I. and that makes sense as a stepping stone in minimizing your future health problems. We were looking for something that also could correct the 20th century nutritional deficiencies that constitute an unrecognized epidemic. We also wanted a modality that could detoxify people as well as a modality that was respectful of biochemical individuality and cognizant of the increasing chemical pollutant load. Macrobiotics was the only thing that answered all of these needs.

Q. Why hasn't my doctor heard of macrobiotics?
A. He's peddling as fast as he can. Give the guy a break. In this era there are over 2000 scientific journals to be read. Our input of information has become staggeringly impossible to be of practical use. Why not give him a copy of this book and make it easy on him. Why should he have to spend years "rediscovering the wheel"?

Q. How can I have rice for breakfast?
A. Just as easily as you can have coffee decaffeinated with trichloroethylene, loaded with pesticides, a devitalized sugary donut made from bleached wheat with many additives, or toast made from the same thing, or orange juice from dyed oranges, heavily pesticided throughout their growth cycle. When you think about it, the English breakfast of baked beans or even kippers is far healthier. Basically you want whole foods that are not devitalized and that have a life force or energy still residing in them.

Q. I've heard you can get really sick if you go off macrobitics.

A.   After 5 1/2 months of macro, I found myself
thousands of miles from home in a remote area.
After a few days I decided to abandon the hope
of continuing macrobiotics while on this trip.
At first I tried to eat cautiously, but after
a week, my old eating habits were in full
swing.

The first thing I noticed was that these old
favorites didn't taste as good anymore, and I
really yearned for some pure G, G and B
(grains, greens and beans). I also felt like
these foods weren't digesting. One day I
decided to try a dish of ice cream and
succumbed to a three hour deep sleep. A few
days later the same treat only caused a 2 hour
nap. I was beginning to adapt (masking).

By the end of a week, I had a night of such
diarrhea that I didn't have two contiguous
hours of sleep. That did it! The hotel would
not locate any brown rice for us and they
would not even cook it if we brought it to
them. There was no alternative. My husband
and I set out to purchase a single electric
burner. The fifth store we consulted had one
for $20. Then we sought out the town's only
health food store and got brown rice, kale,
onions, carrots, Mt. Valley glass bottled
spring water, miso and umeboshi (plums). I
felt like we had discovered gold. Back at the
hotel, I had a sudden blinding headache, and
discovered they had started painting the
elevator next to our room while we were
shopping. We packed and moved. Once we were
resettled, I unpacked my other purchases: a
covered saucepan, knife, spoon, dish and set
to work. In less than 24 hours I was feeling
great again. The experience taught me several
useful lessons:
     1.   I'm no where near ready to expand my
           diet.

2. Macrobiotics is indeed a powerful
    healing tool for my body.
3. I'll not dream of venturing away from
    home without all the supplies to
    provide my own food.
4. When pressed, we can all accomplish
    amazing feats. I must admit, I'm not
    the problem solver, my husband is.
    Had I been alone, I probably would
    have suffered the symptoms. He, on
    the other hand, is not restricted by
    convention and the impossible. He
    sees every obstacle as a tool for
    further growth. It's only too
    logical to him that if G, G and B are
    what I need to feel better, then
    that's precisely what I should have.

    Don't lose sight of the fact that
    negativity and "it's impossible", and
    "I can't" may be part of your
    symptoms too. Actually, as I've
    lectured over the globe, I met many
    orientals who cooked in their hotel
    rooms. And when the restauranteurs
    realize there is a profit to be made
    by just having some healthful, whole
    unbroken grains on the menu, we will
    no longer need to carry these
    supplies.

I realize how absurd our world has gotten
when I'm ecstatic just thinking of finding a
hotel whose guest room windows open and that
serves glass bottled spring water and organic
brown rice.

Q. Why do some people have worse reactions than
    they used to once they veer from macrobiotics?
A. They are unmasked. If your body doesn't like
    something it gives you a symptom. Many people

ignore it or drug it. Once you're on clean whole foods and start eating junk again, you should feel wretched, as I did. If you persist, however, you can adapt again (but you'll develop other problems). When we give a baby processed food, he spits it back in our faces. We think it's cute and ignore the poor kid and force it down him until he adapts.

Q. Is it alright if I eat.......?
A. Remember there are 3 diets. A transition (to ease you into macro), healing (individually prescribed and temporarily restricted) and maintenance (full of variety and fun). The maintenance is most liberal (once you're clear of symptoms, unmasked and unmedicated). The healing diet is the most restricted and it's phases are tailor made to your disease, your general condition, and your monitored response. To plea bargain for foods is to retard your progress. Why not be as strict as necessary and get on with healing, for later you can eat as you want.

Q. I went macro years ago and they made me worse.
A. That's because some counselors may be less experienced or rigid or have not yet adapted to the needs of E.I. The gestalt psychiatrist thinks gestalt psychotherapy is going to help every patient. The Freudian psychiatrist thinks likewise for Freudian analysis, the rational emotive therapist..etc. People get stuck in their own niches where they get the best results. You can't treat a cancer patient the same as an E.I. patient, and further there is tremendous individual variation among people with the same diagnosis. In general, many allergic people do not tolerate grains, especially wheat, nor soy, or ferments. Adaptation must be allowed for.

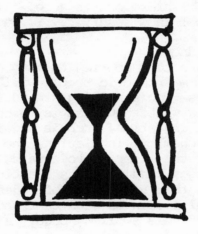

If lack of time is your excuse for quitting, why not read Alan Lakein's classic time management book, <u>How</u> <u>to</u> <u>Get</u> <u>Control</u> <u>of</u> <u>Your</u> <u>Time</u> <u>and</u> <u>Life</u>.

Q. When I'm out of town why don't I just go to a Japanese restaurant?
A. Japanese and Chinese restaurants are just about as far removed from macro as the standard American restaurant. Most all of them use devitalized, bleached white rice and much MSG (which tastes peculiar when you're unmasked). My husband ordered sushi for me on our flight, thinking it resembled my nori rolls; I broke out in song, "If you knew sushi, like I know sushi........."

Q. What is hardness?
A. Hardness is a term applied to many of your organs that macrobiotic people will use. When they diagnose you as having a hard liver, for example, what they mean is through years of much yin ingestion, such as sugars or alcohol or chemical inhalation, the yin response of the liver is to expand, become swollen, boggy, and lose its elasticity. Couple with that your years of ingestion of fats and salts such as much beef and hard cheeses, and this swollen, boggy, expanded liver becomes filled with mucus and fats which block or impede the energy flow. It can also become a breeding ground for chronic infection. Eventually, it can even calcify, especially if you ingest synthetic vitamin D2 enriched products such as milk. It becomes firmer (hence, hardness) until it is very ill and starts adversely affecting other areas of the body.

Q. What is discharge?
A. Discharge is a phenomenon whereby as weight is lost, the pH becomes more balanced and mucus, and old chemicals and toxins are presumably pulled out of hard organs and discharged. There comes a time when many of the stored chemicals and toxins are mobilized and float freely in the bloodstream, thereby mimicking

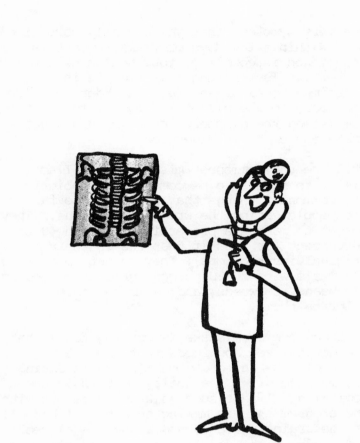

We need good scientific documentation of the effects of macrobiotics. We need to show that you really do detoxify, and correct your nutrient levels. And as we collate this data, we will be able to present it in a way that the scientific medical community can appreciate.

the very symptoms that you normally complained
of. Within a few days or weeks, when this
phenomenon is complete, your health will be
at new levels. During this time it is
sometimes necessary to fast in order to allow
your body to use all of its energy for
completing the discharge phenomenon and not
waste any of it in digestion.

Q. What are the commonest mistakes that I am
likely to make as a newcomer to macrobiotics?
A. The commonest things that I've seen so far
are people eating the wrong proportions. They
forget to make the proportion of grain 40 to
60 percent (or less if that was in their
original instructions). They forget to balance
the meals with 20-30 percent greens and add in
the beans, seaweeds, and ferments (once they
tolerate them).

A second common mistake is getting foods that
are devitalized and foods that are not
organic. The third common mistake is eating
too much food. I was guilty of this in the
beginning. I felt such an urge to get on with
the program that in making sure that I had all
of the grains, greens, and beans, (sea) weeds
and seeds, roots and "fruits", I had enormous
quantities of food at each meal. Fourth is
forgetting to listen to your body. Eat only
when you're hungry. Give it a rest and let it
decide for you when it needs sustenance.
Fifth is neglecting to follow-up in the office
to graduate to the next stage of wellness.

Q. What are some of the reasons for discontinuing
macrobiotics?
A. People who have discontinued give the
following excuses: They didn't have time to
plan, shop, and prepare for the meals. Their
spouse hated the stuff. They didn't like the

One of my goals is to remove the isolation
that people with E.I. and on macro feel. Making
our successes known in the medical literature
should bring us closer to a day when you can go
into any restaurant and have a choice of macro
(just as you now can have special foods for
diabetes or high cholesterol).

259

smells in the house. They found it very
boring. It didn't taste good. It limited
their social lives. However, bear in mind
that if the norm in a restaurant was that you
could find macrobiotic food, it certainly
would change things immensely in many of
those categories. Also, many of those
categories reflect that the person has not had
adequate training in cooking lessons, which
are essential.

Q. What can I drink?
A. Thirst, like any symptom, is a God-given
mechanism for survival. When an animal needs
water, it has thirst and searches for water.
Man cannot rely on this, because (1) he eats
highly salty and fatty foods so he has
abnormal thirst and overworks his kidneys by
drinking to excess. (2) Man drinks for taste
and mood, not for thirst. He drinks because
he likes the sweetness and the high from a
coke. He has distorted his thirst feedback
mechanism.

If one is eating whole grains, greens and
beans, they contain over 50% water and very
little else is needed, especially when salt
is as reduced as it should be. So drink an
occasional cup of tea if you need it. Bancha,
safflower, or roasted barley are fine. Be
sure to use glass bottled spring or well water
for all your cooking and teas, however.

Q. What if I can't give up coffee, cigarettes, or
beer?
A. You are not getting enough bitter greens.
These are bitter cravings and designate the
need for greens and to cut back on salt and
increase the sweets and/or sour.

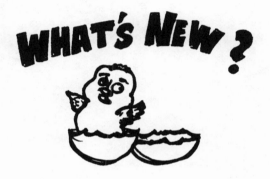

Please check back with the office at least yearly, even if it's just by mail. There is constant newness. By knowing what your current status of gains and problems is, we can help you in your quest for wellness.

WRITE YOUR QUESTIONS AND COMMENTS DOWN NOW WHILE
YOU'RE THINKING OF THEM.......

CHAPTER IX

WHAT NOW?

As you can see I've tried to accomplish a number of items.

(1) Top priority is to get people who are still suffering from chronic diseases, especially E.I. and Candida, better. (By now you realize that nearly all chronic disease and Candida is E.I.)

(2) Help others who are not getting as much out of life as they could to find a new level of wellness. And, to prevent future disease.

(3) Be open minded about a non-medical discipline yet at the same time maintain some semblance of scientific credibility.

(4) Give credit to macrobiotics for this massive contribution.

However, I cannot at this stage support all that macrobiotics stands for.

(1) People have developed and died from cancer while on macrobiotics. Like anything else there are no guarantees, except death and taxes.

(2) There are many strange sounding remedies like taping an ume plum to your navel for sea sickness, baking some of your hair and making a tea for uterine hemorrhaging. Some leaders have recommended you eat only one apple a year, condone wife beating, and denigrate women with hairy legs!

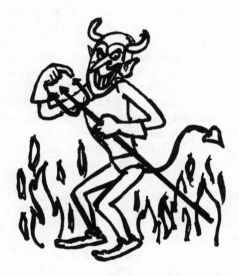

    As with every new and controversial endeavor,
you want to play the devil's advocate and look
objectively at both sides (yin and yang?).

(3)   How can I justify referring some of my
        sickest patients to a counselor who has
        absolutely no medical training, possibly not
        even a high school education and maybe a
        week's crash course somewhere. There's no
        gold standard by which we can measure
        competency in macrobiotic diagnosis and
        counseling. I guess if you wanted to be
        safe you'd go to Michio Kushi in Brookline
        Massachusetts. But I've taken care of
        patients who went there and were failures
        and eventually flew to Syracuse for
        treatment instead. I'm not knocking them.
        I'm sure they have healed failures of mine.
        I'm pointing out legitimate problems. I
        would like to see macrobiotics attain enough
        credibility that an institute such as Mr.
        Kushi's reaches a level of acceptance by the
        medical profession. This would entail a
        standard of excellence that we could count
        on as in any other medical specialty. This
        can only happen, as I see it, through
        scientific study.

Now this will make many people in macrobiotics
very angry for just as in medicine, there are
people who feel you must be all or nothing. They
arrogantly feel you should be a total devotee of
macrobiotics in every phase of your life. They
resent their diet being used for its own sake and
even prophesies that it won't work without the
whole philosophy. The problem is just as with yin
and yang, nothing is absolute. And by the way, no
two books can ever agree on that! Something as
fundamental as what is yin and what is yang is
fraught with controversy. Even Ohsawa called
things yin in the seventies that years earlier he
had called yang.

Isn't it ironic--all we ever wanted was
health. When medicine couldn't give it to us, we

found answers in ecology. Then doctors and insurance companies got nasty because we were forced to look for wellness outside of their system. They wanted us to get well through their system.

Now we've found another aid, macrobiotics, and we'll probably have more people angry with us for not totally embracing their system. When will the world recognize biochemical individuality and allow us to freely pick and choose (while monitoring our bodies' responses) the best of all worlds for ourselves!

Since I wear three hats (conventional medicine, environmental medicine and macrobiotics), let's look at some of the most salient difficulties with macrobiotic philosophy.

(1) It has many contradictions. They even have experts arguing whether a new food is yin or yang.

(2) They reversed the Chinese definition of yin and yang, which adds to the confusion. Fortunately descriptive terms, expansive and contractive have supplemented.

(3) Alkaline and acid do not directly apply to yin and yang. Furthermore, many sources disagree as to which foods fall into which categories. Even within the same work there are contradictions. For example, Aihara's classic Acid and Alkaline classifies azuki and tofu as yin acid forming (pg 90), but alkaline forming (pg 38, 39); confusing for the neophyte. A clearer treatise of these issues is needed if macro is to grow into a self-help discipline as it espouses.

(4) It gets too confusing as one is taught that processes of food preparation can alter the yin or yang properties of a food.

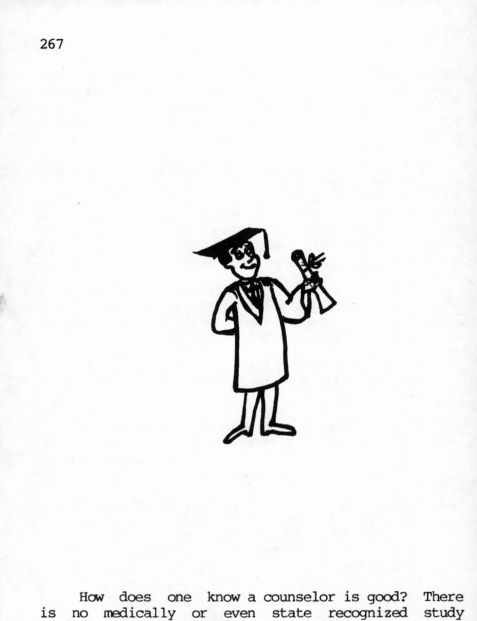

How does one know a counselor is good? There is no medically or even state recognized study program with certification. It takes the Chinese years to learn oriental diagnosis, but westerners can take 1-6 weeks of a course and call themselves counselors. There does not appear to be a governing/regulatory board.

(5) After reading over two dozen macrobiotics
works, there are many unanswered questions and
no recognized authority to consult.

On the other hand, there are many extremely
helpful ideas that emerge from these works. So
where do we go from here?

———— ———— ———— ———— ———— ———— ————

The discipline of macrobiotics is so
comprehensive that many books must be consulted. A
major text is in need, where important facts are
collated. For example:

Did You Know?

that wakame seaweed has more B12 than beef or
 pork?

that Kombu has twice as much B12 as eggs?

that broccoli, brussel sprouts, collard greens,
 mustard greens and parsley have more vitamin
 C than oranges?

that millet has almost twice the iron as beef?

that Kale has twice as much calcium as cheese?

that sesame seeds have more calcium than milk?

that ume plums have more calcium, iron, and
 phosphorus than apples, strawberries, or
 peaches?

that ume plums are excellent alkalinizers as well
 as being neutralizers of toxins and lactic
 acid (They work best for yin (sweets/alcohol)
 hangovers, while apple cider/Kuzu or
 scallion/miso soup works better for yang
 (meat/salt) hangovers). Umeboshi is 20% salt,
 so limit to one a day.

that miso, tamari, and gomashio also help to
    neutralize symptoms from excessive smoke
    exposure? The first two are 13-18% salt so
    limit them, especially when in the healing
    mode.

that if you are caught out eating fish without any
    daikon or ume, you could order horseradish
    along with it?

that miso soup with scallion or barley are good to
    reduce the symptoms from meat?

that grated daikon and ginger help mobilize sticky
    mucous?

that cravings for coffee, beer, or cigarettes
    (bitter) can be helped by increasing your
    (bitter) greens?

that sweet cravings can be overcome with sweet
    grains and vegetables like sweet rice or your
    squash soup?

that too much sour can be counteracted by pungent
    (ginger)?

that	sour	counters	pungent (ginger)
"	bitter	"	salty
"	pungent	"	bitter (greens)
"	salty	"	sweet
"	sweet	"	sour, etc?

that one tbs. sesame seeds has more calcium than
    one cup of milk?

that millet, chickpeas, or lentils have more iron
    than beef liver?

Why are vitamin levels needed if this diet is so healthy? With a diet of predominantly cooked foods, there can be a shortage of vitamins that are destroyed by heat, like B, or C.

Rationale for Remedies

What factors contribute the worst to acidity?

1. Poor nutritional status from depleted soils, non-organic foods, processed foods and poor eating habits all stress the chemistry and push it to find compensatory routes.

2. An overloaded chemical environment causes stress to the xenobiotic detoxication system, through the formation of free radicals, which are crazy unfocused electrons that destroy cell membranes and initiate disease, increase and add to the acidity and biochemical stress.

3. A poorly balanced diet with emphasis on sweets and meats creates a high acid stress.

4. Unhealthy thoughts like anger, worry, jealousy, fear, hate, and resentment cause the release of brain neurotransmitters which in turn trigger the release of hormones and peptides that add to the acidity to be neutralized by the body. More importantly, these emotions indicate there is imbalance (they are a symptom) which needs to be addressed.

Why is acidity bad?

Increased acid is the antagonist to good health. The body must constantly work to keep it in check. Likewise, increased alkalinity could create uncontrolled cravings or an extreme feeling of unwellness until it is corrected.

Acidity pulls calcium from bones so that early dental and jaw bone disease results with eventual false teeth. Acidity uses up magnesium so cardiac arrhythmia and neck and back muscle spasms occur more easily with seemingly minor triggers. Or other smooth muscles go into spasm easily resulting in diarrhea, migraine, or asthma.

Although few sources agree, a rough approximation of foods (and drink and chemicals) can be categorized as I have portrayed them in the diagram (p. 275). By studying this and the many texts that go into greater detail, you can begin to appreciate how you can manipulate your body chemically with what you choose to eat. You are like a perpetual laboratory experiment. You can control your health, your moods, and your energy by just observing and listening to the feedback. Isn't it exciting?

Acid and Alkaline, Yin and Yang, Expansive and Contractive

In order to heal the quickest it seems logical to take as much extraneous work away from the body as possible. After all, when you have a fever and pneumonia you don't dig ditches, you go to bed.

Since the body works hard at keeping the pH or hydrogen ion content at 7.43, it seems logical to eat near this with 50:50 whole grains and veggies as opposed to two colas and a candy bar.

And so the pH or acid/alkaline content of foods has been determined. It has another benefit because it helps you determine what to take to balance a craving. For example if you've had an ice cream and feel sleepy and moody, try some ume plums to alkalinize your system.

Yin and yang are part of the oriental philosophy of opposites. They apply to every force of life and help establish our concept of balance. Everything has some yin and some yang qualities. Nothing is totally one or the other. Furthermore, the yinness or yangness of something is relative to everything else. Nothing stands alone.

We have modern sayings that express the duality of life and remind us to always look for the balance ("Every cloud has a silver lining,"). And one of the seven laws of the Order of the Universe according to macrobiotic philosophy is "That which has a beginning has an end." That might be analogous to "It's always darkest before the dawn".

When yin and yang are applied to food, however, the picture becomes complicated. Acid and alkaline content can be measured in a laboratory. Yin and yang cannot. Not only that but some people spend their lives arguing over what is yin or yang.

To further complicate matters, what Mr. Ohsawa called yin in 1928, he called yang in his 1960 writings. Yin and yang are also relative. A chicken is yang compared with fish, but is yin compared with salt.

George Ohsawa's terms expansive and contractive seem to handle our needs better. Although there is no across the board correlation, in general foods that are acid are also yin or expansive. Likewise, foods that are alkaline are often contractive or yang. You will find many exceptions to these however.

In general, contractiveness has features of being low growing, slow growing, and hard, needing long cooking. Yang alkaline foods include Bancha tea, dandelion tea, lotus root, burdock root, sesame and soy sauce, miso, salt, and umeboshi. Yang acid-forming foods include grains, fish, fowl, beef and eggs.

Yang foods tend to warm the body. Too much yang leads to contractive symptoms such as arthritis, aggression, inflexibility and arrogance. These can be modified to good qualities of moral strength.

Expansiveness represents features of high growing, quick growing, soft, growing in a warm climate, being watery and big, and requiring little or no cooking. Yin alkalinizing foods include honey, coffee, herb tea, spices, seeds, vegetables, and some beans. Yin acid-forming substances include chemicals, medications, sugar, alcohol, some beans, oils and nuts.

The expansive foods tend to cool the body. The symptoms of over expansiveness can be allergies, hypersensitivity, spaciness, confusion, and inability to concentrate. These can be modified to bring out one's artistic and creative nature.

Isn't it interesting that this ages old philosophy describes our 21st century disease of E.I. perfectly?

But should this all sound a bit confusing, remember there are no absolutes. Nothing is totally yin or yang. Everything has aspects of both, although one predominates. And these qualities in everything are relative to other things. Nor are yin and yang good or bad. They are in fact complimentary........the spice of life.

275

Very roughly speaking, acid/alkaline,
expansive/contractive and yin/yang
could look somewhat like this:

Yin acid	Expansive	Yin alkaline
chemicals		wine, colas
drugs, medicines		lemon, yogurt, ginger
sugar, candy		coffee, mineral water
vinegar		raisins, bananas
whiskey, beer		shitake, cinnamon
olive oil, sesame oil		apple, cherries
almonds, tofu		cabbage, broccoli
chickpeas		pumpkin, onion
azuki		daikon, nori, hiziki
tofu		

CENTER

		seeds, squash
	macaroni	carrots,
		milk
	oats	kuzu tea
	barley	burdock, kombu
	rice, wheat	millet
	white fish	lotus
	fowl	dandelion, mu tea
	meat	gomashio, soy sauce
	tuna, salmon	wakame
	eggs	miso, ume, salt
	ginseng	

Yang acid	Contractive	Yang alkaline

As you see, the more extreme foods are at the ends, as far from the center as possible. You can easily appreciate how a specified amount of a food could be therapeutic but why an excess would help to create further imbalance. Your best guide is to listen to your unmasked body.

Basically you want to do the majority of your eating near the center or fulcrum of the balance scale. But when imbalance occurs, you can see what remedy would most likely correct it or bring you closer to the center again.

Clearly, by beginning to understand the acid/alkali format, you can understand why certain remedies work. Just don't go out on the ends away from the fulcrum unless you are in great health or it's a time for a festival. The majority of the time you want to give your body the room it needs to heal.

Say you've overdosed on sweets, or you have a craving for chocolate? Miso soup or umeboshi (plums) may take care of that for you. I use mustard greens (because I loved bitter chocolate) in chickpea miso soup, some barley (for the calories and hunger), and sprinkle gomashio over the top (for the crunchies). You could dangle bittersweet chocolate under my nose and I have no craving. I know it sounds bizarre because when I first tested umeboshi (plums), for example, I was sure everyone who used them was nuts. But once you establish balance and see how soothing it feels, you will learn to listen to your body and correct its imbalances. Remember, a craving is merely a transient chemical imbalance and with thoughtless binges you overcorrect and use up too much biochemical energy. Also you will shortly have another craving because you have overshot the mark. Giving in to a craving means indulging in an extreme food that throws you past the fulcrum to the opposite end of the scale.

In essence, when you are balanced, you feel satiated and comfortable and are not driven to eat in excess. Right now Americans have such distorted tastebuds and body feedback/recognition systems that they eat only for taste and mood.

Say you have diarrhea, a very yin (expansive) symptom -- you could turn it off with a seaweed soup with miso, or kuzu/umeboshi/soy sauce/bancha tea.

Or say you overdosed on meat; grated daikon with a few drops of soy sauce will bring you back to the center. Carrot or apple juice can also do the trick.

So you logically ask, why don't I balance meat with wine? And obviously many cultures do so and quite healthfully. But then you are pushing the extremes of the balance beam -- something you want to save for when you are healthy. The further from the fulcrum, the more biochemical energy that will be needed to establish balance. And you're trying to reserve all of your energy for healing at this point in time.

I did well for a long time on sugar, wine, cheese, and meat. The body breakdown steadily progressed, but I was able to keep up by increasing my drugs for pain and other symptoms. Then when the systems finally collapsed, I had multiple target organ involvement, and I had exhausted my wad of medicines. That's the time that a massive diet and lifestyle change (environmental controls, assess thoughts and goals) becomes necessary. That's when a plethora of nutritional deficiencies must be sought and corrected: meticulous attention to diet, nutritional status, environment, and the psyche is required.

In the preceding macrobiotic scheme, it looks as though milk should be a great buffer, but too many people know it gives them tremendous congestion. Likewise many Candida and mold sensitive people cannot eat ferments like miso until they have been on the restricted macro diet for a few months.

Now you can begin to see how futile most diets are in helping weight loss, because cravings are not neutralized. For example, high meat (acid, contractive) creates a craving for the opposite for balance, hence alcohol and sugar (expansive) and/or coffee (alkaline). And likewise those who eat a large amount of fruits (expansive, alkaline) in the name of dieting, foster balancing cravings of salty foods (contractive), sweets (acid), and meat (contractive, acid). Now you can see also why diets that rely on one kind of food are destined to fail in the long run.

Hunger after a meal most likely indicates imbalance; for starters, often it's time to abandon supplements. Next hunger can signify the need for protein foods or broken grains. Perhaps assimilation is poor. Lack of joy and rigidity may indicate too much of one cooking style, or too much cooked food in general. Raw foods possess a life force that is destroyed by cooking.

It also appears on the chart that a diet balanced in sugar-coffee-meat and salt should make one feel pretty good, and indeed there are many healthy people who eat just that way. So why is it that some of us do so much better with grains and greens? It seems that biochemical individuality reigns over everything including macrobiotics.

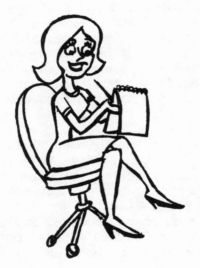

Even though they are not certified, there are several good counselors in our area. Since they don't send referral letters like physicians do you'll need to send me an audio tape of your consultation if you want us to be a part of your care.

In the words of David Yarrow,
Health is balance, and sickness is imbalance. Our medicine is simply the way we live. The mind and body are complementary and form a unified whole. They are yin and yang. Problems in either will create distress and disorder in the opposite.

Nearly everyone with E.I. has a severe acid - alkaline imbalance. Not only are most too acidic, but their ability to neutralize and remove acid is severely disturbed and exhausted. Two primary alkalinizing minerals in the body are sodium and calcium. Today many people rely on heavy doses of salt and dairy to alkalinize the acid (or meats, sweets and processed foods). Many stones (and arteriosclerotic deposits) result form insoluble mineral salts condensing in the kidneys, gall bladder, (and blood vessels). Fresh vegetables (from sea and land) are the primary alkalinizing foods. Whole grains are next, with much individual variation. Thorough chewing alkalinizes whole grains. Kuzu-umeboshi tea can provide fast relief for many acid conditions from sour stomach to fatigue.

Mucous is a general term for the waste and debris in the system. Dairy, oils, sugar, and baked flour products are the primary offenders. This excess mucous can eventually be eliminated through the intestine with a macrobiotic diet of whole grains and vegetables. Onion, daikon, cruciferae, garlic and barley are among the foods that can help in dissolving this material. Seaweeds are a vital source of precious balanced minerals to strengthen the body buffering fluids. White ginger, exercise and skin brushing help to stimulate the circulation.

For all its strangeness, inconsistencies and drawbacks, macrobiotics has the potential to turn around our present epidemic in disguise of subclinical malnutrition. It also has the potential to arrest and even reverse a vast amount of degenerative disease (which this subclinical malnutrition has contributed to). Macrobiotics also embraces the reality that we are a part of the macro and micro cosmos. When this is realized, it makes it difficult for an intelligent person to knowingly pollute his body with inferior food, pesticides, additives and drugs and to pollute his environment with acid rain, nuclear and chemical wastes. On the home front he will opt for a chemically less-contaminated lifestyle as well.

By checking for nutrient (vitamin, mineral, essential fatty acid, amino acid) balance, we hope to maximize wellness and further substantiate the benefits of macrobiotics. By documenting the discharge phenomenon (liver functions, monitoring depurated xenobiotics) we are trying to establish a scientific rationale for macrobitics. Then, and only then can medical acceptance come about, which in turn should lead to wider acceptance and availability of wholesome foods on airlines and in restaurants. The global benefits are awesome.

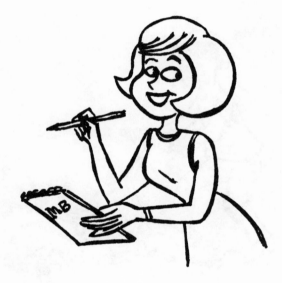

Don't forget to bring both questionnaires, filled out beforehand, to every visit. Otherwise we'll have to spend time asking you all those background questions and won't have time for the actual consultation.

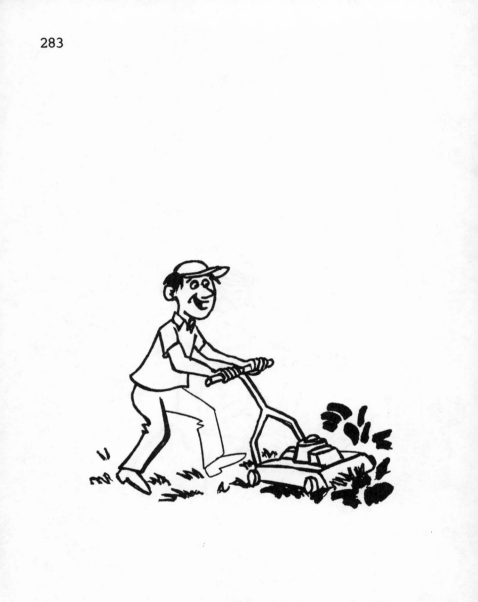

Most people have spouses who mow the lawn. My poor husband can usually find his wife grazing on the lawn, instead. I eat most of my dandelions.

Biochemical Blunders:
The Innocence of Medicine?

In the following table which compares the philosophy of conventional medicine with that of macrobiotics and environmental medicine, it can be seen how naive conventional medicine is. Is this true innocence or waiting for the impossible, yet eternal dream of double blind proof? The FDA usually requires double blind proof which works for drugs and surgeries, but not lifestyle changes. With a new drug you give 100 people the real thing and 100 people a dummy capsule. The physician and patients are unaware of which anyone is receiving until the study is over (hence double blind).

It seems that the environmental approach is so logical that the only dissenters that will remain are those motivated by ego and money before health.

I don't mean to place blame anywhere, and certainly not with the overworked, over harassed physician. The poor guy studied diligently and works his best to apply what he learned in medical school. Somewhere along the line in our training though, respect for biochemical individuality and ecologically sound lifestyles was lost. Instead we capriciously pollute our food, air and water and when this causes symptoms we use drugs to suppress them.

Fortunately, environmental, nutritional, biochemical, and toxicologic research has accumulated sufficient data to usher in a more responsible era. A renaissance in medicine is here.

View On	As seen by Conventional Medicine	Environmental Medicine and Macrobiotics
Drugs	a necessary part of overcoming illness	rarely necessary if a healthy body is maintained with chemically clean air, food and water.
Illness	seen as bad, requiring drugs to suppress symptoms	seen as good; an opportunity to cleanse, identify and correct an imbalance
Environment	something to be manipulated, fought and changed to suit our whims	an irreplaceable resource to be appreciated and continue to adapt to and live with in harmony
People	all the same	no two alike due to biochemical individuality
Medicine	cookbook style	individualized

Vitamins	not needed in general	crucial to replace through whole foods and/or supplements, deficiencies due to processed foods and the current extra stress on detoxification systems
Processed Foods	many healthy people live on them	undesirable, studies support inferior nutrition
Diet	very little influence over medical conditions	a major determiner of health
Health	absence of diagnosable disease	looking, feeling and performing great
Diagnosis of Disease	mostly through documentation of abnormal blood test, culture, physical abnormality, or X-ray	consists of any symptom that inhibits the maximum wellness
Masking	non-existent	once you're eating well, your body alarms ring (symptoms) when you eat something that it doesn't like or need (until it becomes adapted and then the alarm is muted)

Adaptation	inconsequential	the price to be paid for chronic adaptation is chronic disease
Cravings	silly, meaningless whimsical	an important symptom of bio-chemical imbalance
Control of Health	lies with the physician	lies with the individual, physician is the consultant
Treatment	all people with the same disease should have the same treatment	treatment is individual, no two people are alike
Minor Complaints (ie: fatigue)	usually due to hypochondrasis, stress or depression	a symptom of biochemical imbalance; an early warning of more severe disease to come
Aging	unchangeable	some genetic control but also the total accumulation of free radical destruction mediated by chronic overcompensation and adaptation to environment

Individual Person	a clone of every-one else	each one bio-chemically unique: one man's meat is another man's poison or to put it macro-biotically, one man's weeds are another man's dinner
Chronic Degenerative Disease	to be expected and and accepted; unavoidable	having an environmental trigger, abnormal and controllable
Relation of Man to Environment	little bearing on health, except for a few recognized occupational diseases	a major factor that cannot be ignored if well-ness is to be attained.

The naivete of medicine when it comes to nutritional matters is startling in view of its fantastic accomplishments in other areas.

Take these four simple examples:
(1) The calcium craze. Doctors have recommended everything from antacids to bone meal, without a thought of the need to balance this calcium carefully with other nutrients. And cognizance for the causes is not appreciated. If one reads the biochemistry literature it's quite apparent that processed foods are high in phosphates. Phosphates in turn inhibit the absorption of calcium.

Also a high acid diet (processed foods, sweets, meats) uses up calcium as a buffer, stealing it from the bone. And if zinc, magnesium, boron, manganese and other trace elements are deficient, as they commonly are due to processed foods and devitalized soils, then calcium cannot be incorporated into bone. As far as supplementation goes, hypochlorhydria (low stomach acid) and antacids inhibit absorption and many recommended forms of calcium have very poor absorption to begin with. And again, if the status of the accessory minerals are not known and adjusted, there will be limited incorporation of the calcium into bone.

(2) The cholesterol controversy. Doctors recommend diets of plastic foods (artificial eggs, butters, sausages), and dangerous trans fatty acids (margarine, processed foods, polyunsaturated vegetable oils) that promote free radical damage (degenerative disease, allergies, cancer). When that fails, they prescribe cholesterol-lowering drugs that also inhibit the uptake of important nutrients. Don't forget, when you're nutrient depleted, the last thing you want is another drug that further depletes.

(3) Alzheimer's disease. Billions of dollars are spent yearly on sustaining victims of this disease. But where is the education of doctors and the public to reduce their intake of aluminum? How many people use aluminum cookware, antacids, douches, deodorants and foods? Aluminum is in many processed foods (salt, flours, baking powder, cheeses, beer) as an anti-caking agent. Plus undetected calcium, zinc or magnesium deficiencies allow aluminum to be deposited more easily in the brain.

(4) Unrecognized zinc deficiency. The literature supports the presence of a silent epidemic of zinc deficiency. Yet an rbc zinc is not part of a routine chemical profile. No foods are fortified with zinc (except a few baby formulas). And yet it's crucial in every metabolic pathway of the body and a deficiency can help promote cancer, AIDS, chemical intolerance, other nutritional deficiencies and more.

Those were just four simple examples of current medical problems that could be corrected by just avoiding a processed foods diet. And left unchecked, each one can cause severely debilitating chronic symptoms. How very cost effective it would be to educate people about the value of eating whole foods and checking a simple rbc zinc blood test. But first the medical school curriculum must teach the biochemistry of nutrition and environmental medicine.

There is already a plethora of evidence. On one hand we have a silent epidemic of malnutrition that contributes to chronic degenerative illness. And on the other, we have a diet of whole foods with a great track record for healing the impossible. What are we waiting for?

We've distorted our precious feedback system by eating processed foods. We crave sweets, fats, salts, and drinks. We overwork the gastrointestinal tract, liver and kidneys as well as plug arteries and put on unwanted weight.

Worst of all, we suffer anger, jealousy, depression, aggression, and self-pity. Don't forget, if you're standing on one leg, it's easier to knock you over. Well, if you're not playing with a full deck of nutrients, it's easier to create disease in you. And disease is not limited to physical symptoms. When you're not biochemically balanced, it's easy for seemingly inconsequential triggers to throw you into a rage. Remember just a zinc deficiency alone can affect a number of brain chemicals and neurotransmitters that control happy moods and stability. Mood swings, unhappiness and lack of enthusiasm are symptoms.

Likewise faulty neurotransmitters that result can further distort the system. This in turn can lead to increased vulnerability, reactions, and symptoms, many of which are cerebral. It's a vicious cycle or a downward spiral that can lead to poor learning ability, poor social skills, poor school and work performances, delinquency and crime. The handwriting is on the wall.

Likewise, bad chemistry coupled with bad food and environment accelerates aging. In biochemical terms, aging is nothing more than free radical attack on cell membranes resulting in loss of flexibility. Inflexible cell membranes can lead to swelling or heart problems, arteriosclerosis, senility and organ damage. The body becomes inflexible as does the mind. In fact that may be the problem with our detractors.

A 1987 survey of 11,000 people by the National Cancer Institute in Washington concluded that 80% of the 11,000 people interviewed never ate whole grains. Other than potatoes and salad, 49% never ate vegetables. Another 40% never had a daily fruit. But 40% had daily nitrate-containing bacon or luncheon meat.

In the same year, the director of the Division of Cancer Prevention and Control for NCI stated at a Florida conference, "There is now general scientific evidence that about 80% of cancer cases appear to be linked to the way people live their lives. The role of diet in the cause and prevention of cancer is particularly important". Too bad it took until 1987 to figure this out. Others have known it for decades.

The bottom line is that environmental medicine coupled with macrobiotics is light years ahead of conventional medicine in terms of chronic disease. On the other hand, conventional medicine cannot be surpassed in it's handle on acute disease. It's time for a marriage of the two. The stormy courtship is over.

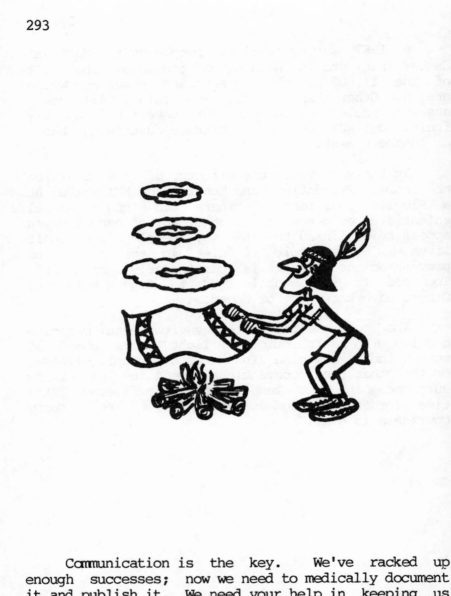

Communication is the key. We've racked up enough successes; now we need to medically document it and publish it. We need your help in keeping us posted on your progress. Blood tests are useful to document discharge and improvement in nutrient levels.

As a specialist in environmental medicine who is on the leading edge (which also means the firing line!) I am grateful for all that my illness has taught me, and for all that my patients have taught me. I am grateful for all the discoveries of biochemists and toxicologists around the world (however incredibly ignored they may be by the medical profession) and I am grateful for macrobiotics and the people who brought it to us. In order to return that gratitude I think macrobiotics deserves more careful study and documentation so that we may give a gift in return; widespread acceptance and appreciation of its principles. For you now can appreciate more than ever that you have great control through foods, over your health and your moods. Truly, YOU ARE WHAT YOU ATE.

PUBLISHED
PAPERS

Case Studies

RESISTANT CASES: RESPONSE TO MOLD IMMUNOTHERAPY AND ENVIRONMENTAL AND DIETARY CONTROLS

Sherry A. Rogers, MD, FACA, FAAEM*

KEY WORDS

Mold spores
Allergy
Immunotherapy
Fungi

ABSTRACT

Diverse recalcitrant allergic symptoms may be caused by sensitivity to fungi. In this study patients with symptoms resistant to current therapy, including eczema, hyperactivity, depression, asthma, edema, cystic acne, vasculitis, urticaria, dizziness, migraine, weakness, exhaustion and atopic dermatitis underwent five-fold serial dilution end point titration with 21 different fungal extracts. All fungi were tested individually and some also as components of mixes. If testing with the mix and all of its components produced the same end point for wheal growth, the mix was used therapeutically. If none of the fungal components had the same end point as the entire mix, the positive fungi were given individually. If most of the component fungi had the same end points as the mix, the mix was given. Patients concurrently followed an elimination diet, avoiding common allergenic foods such as milk, wheat, corn and especially foods containing fermentation products, such as bread, cheese, alcohol, vinegar, salad dressing, mayonnaise, ketchup, mustard, chocolate and processed foods. Ten cases are cited, describing significant improvements in symptoms. Symptoms returned with double-blind substitution of saline placebos for treatment injections, and were cleared on reinstitution of treatments. Removal of carpet, washing of surfaces with borax, permeating the home with vinegar and chlorine bleach fumes, and installation of electrostatic precipitators and ultraviolet lights are discussed as ways to reduce indoor fungi.

* Northeast Center for Environmental Medicine, 2800 W. Genesee St., Syracuse, NY 13219

Fungi produce some of the most potent toxins, hallucinogens, and antibiotics known to man and are indispensable to the food industry (1). They can thrive in conditions inimicable to many other living organisms and under certain climatic conditions can produce billions of spores. During the height of the pollen season it is not unusual for the ratio of *Cladosporium* (*Hormodendrum*) spores to pollen to be 1,000:1 (2).

Fungi have been shown to produce symptoms in the allergic individual (3-5). Allergists usually test a patient's degree of sensitivity to the major molds, *Hormodendrum*, *Aspergillus*, *Alternaria* and *Penicillium*, and test a dozen or fewer other fungi on an individual basis.

In a previous study (6) we showed that by substituting a medium of malt agar extract for Sabouraud's medium, by increasing plate exposure time from 10 minutes to 1 hour, and by saving plates for up to three weeks to allow the slow growers to appear, we produced a 32% yield increase for cultured fungi. We then showed that the fungal flora was in a state of constant change, and that for best results gravity plates should be placed during periods of human activity, between knee and shoulder height (7). A third paper gave an updated view of our region's fungal flora (8).

The purpose of the present study was to determine the practical and clinical significance of incorporating fungi we had previously isolated into a scheme for treating a variety of recalcitrant allergic symptoms.

Materials and methods

Twenty-one fungi were selected for this trial and divided into mixes as shown in Table 1.

Table 1.
Components of mold mixes used

Mix A	*Aspergillus, Alternaria, Hormodendrum* (*Cladosporium*), *Penicillium*
Mix B	*Epicoccum, Fusarium, Pullularia* (*Aureobasidium*)
Mix D	*Fomes, Mucor, Phoma, Rhodotorula*
Mix E	*Cephalosporium, Botrytis, Geotrichum, Helminthosporium, Stemphyllium*

Trichophyton, Candida, Epidermophyton, Rhizopus and *Sporobolomyces* were tested individually.

We tested with several different strengths of each fungus to assess the relative degree of sensitivity to each. Five-fold serial dilutions (9) were prepared for each fungus, as described previously for chemical testing (10). Dilution #1 was four parts Hollister-Stier diluent and one part of the concentrate. Dilution #2 was four parts diluent and one part #1, and so on. Intradermal testing began

with an injection of 0.05 ml of #5. Only that amount was injected to produce a 7x7mm wheal. If no wheal growth occurred, 0.05 ml of #4 was applied, and so on until a 2mm wheal growth was obtained. Again, each time only the amount necessary to produce a 7x7mm wheal was injected. The last negative dilution (no wheal growth) which preceded the first positive wheal growth was the treatment dose. If #2 dilution produced no growth, the test was considered negative. If #5 showed 2mm wheal growth, it was considered positive and weaker dilutions were tested until the first negative dilution was found. This first negative was used as the treatment dose.

All fungi were tested individually and as components of the respective mixes. If testing the mix and all of its components produced the same end point for wheal growth, the mix was used therapeutically. If none of the fungal components had the same end point as the entire mix, the positive fungi were given individually. If most of the component fungi had the same end points as the mix, the mix was given.

The mixes were prepared with equal parts of their constituent fungi and serially diluted five-fold just as the individual fungi were, as described above. The dose administered for all antigens was held constant at 0.05cc twice weekly for one month and weekly thereafter. The doses were not raised.

All patients were tested in the winter to avoid pollen exposure. Those sensitive to pollens had them included in their immunotherapy schedules. Likewise, patients shown to be sensitive to housedust and housedust mite *Dermatophagoides pteronyssinus* had those antigens included in their medication.

At the beginning of the test period, patients were placed on a major elimination diet which prohibited such commonly consumed foods as milk, wheat, corn, and ferments (bread, cheese, alchohol, vinegar, salad dressing, mayonnaise, ketchup, mustard, chocolate and processed foods). They were allowed to eat foods they knew to be safe and that they did not normally eat more frequently than once a week.

Results

The following cases represent the results observed in many of over a thousand patients treated in this manner. For brevity, the original cases selected have been reduced.

Case 1—K.W., a 33-year-old male, had facial, arm, torso and leg eczema since childhood. For the previous 11 years he had severe eczema with marked exfoliation of his lichenified skin. He also suffered from chronic diarrhea. He had been thoroughly examined at several major hospitals in the northwest and treated without improvement by four allergists and three dermatologists. He lived in a trailer in the woods and suspected that molds were part of his problem.

Laboratory findings revealed increased T-4 cells of 60.2% (normal 38-53%) and B cells of 18.9% (normal 7-11%), decreased T-8 cells of 10.3% (normal 18-30) and NK cells of 2.1% (normal 6-13%) and IgE of 33,088 I.U. Unlike the typical patient with hyper-IgE syndrome, he had not had so much as a cold in five years. He knew that milk caused severe exfoliation within a day and his milk RAST was moderately positive.

Within 13 days after initiation of therapy his skin was totally cleared by maintaining the elimination diet and receiving his dust, dust mite and mold injections. This was the first time in 11 years that he had been free of eczema, in spite of many medications, including oral steroids, and immunotherapy trials. His IgE went from 33,088 I.U. to 8,809 I.U. after four months and to 6,456 after six months. After one year it was 2,305 I.U., and after 2 years it was 1,321. He has remained clear for over four years. His severe total body eczematous dermatitis recurs with dietary indiscretion or with double-blind substitution of normal saline for his mold-mite-dust injections. (See before and after photos , Figure 1)

Figure 1
Case 1 K.W.

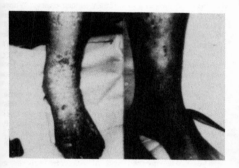

Before immunotherapy   After one month's
                            immunotherapy

Case 2—C.V., a 37-year-old female, had severe facial atopic dermatitis for six years with large erythematous, tender, pruritic papules. Her IgE was unremarkable at 17 I.U. She thought that molds were a problem since her face would burn and tingle when she went outdoors in the fall. Many foods were avoided and the remaining foods rotated on a four day cycle to control symptoms. After receiving injections her facial dermatitis cleared, except when normal saline placebos were substituted double-blind. (Figure 2)

Figure 2
Case 2 C.V.

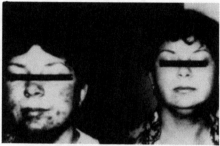

Before immunotherapy   After three month's
                            immunotherapy

Case 3—C.H., an 8-year-old boy, was on 10mg Dexedrine t.i.d. for hyperactivity. He was tested with the fungal extracts and placed on appropriate immunotherapy. Within one month he was able to discontinue the Dexedrine, his attention span improved to the point where he was teachable, his behavior was markedly improved, he grew in height and teeth had erupted after a 2 year arrest.

Before sensitivity testing for molds, he could draw a flower and write his name at a level compatible with his age. Testing with molds reproduced his hyperactivity and his best effort at repeating what he had drawn just five minutes earlier was more compatible with that of a 3-year-old. When the treatment dose was used, his hyperactivity ceased and his writing and drawing returned to normal. (Figure 3)

After four months this boy, who was previously unable to be taught, was earning A's in school. One year later a placebo was substituted for his active medication unbeknown to the allergy nurses administering the injections, to the patient, and to the boy's parents. Within two weeks the mother presented with a black eye the boy had given her for no apparent reason. At that time she stated that his behavior suggested that he was no longer receiving his injections. Also within that two week period two school teachers had gone to the principal and requested that he not be allowed to return the next year. Furthermore, he had been taken by the police to their station twice for discipline after he had come home from school and made calls to the police advising them of non-existent emergencies at his home. When his injections were reinstated, his life returned to normal.

Figure 3
Case 3 C.H.

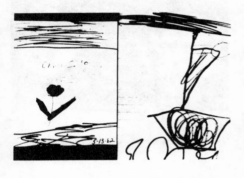

| While being tested with pollen extracts | While being tested with mold extracts* |

* When he was given the neutralizing dose, his drawing returned to normal

Case 4—F.N., a 48-year-old barber, for 6 years had had up to 25 severe headaches a month. They began with the right eye becoming glassy. The right side of his face would swell, the eye would tear, and incapacitating pain would leave him bedridden for two days, contemplating suicide. No amount of analgesics, beta blockers, antihistamines or vasoconstrictors had alleviated the problem. With appropriate injections the headaches ceased. One year later they recurred for the first time, after the injections had been stopped for 10 days.

Case 5—W.B., 41, was a college professor and chairman of his department. Eighteen months prior to his first office visit he developed what he thought was the flu, but it never resolved. He had constant non-vertiginous dizziness, headache, and incapacitating

weakness that would fluctuate in intensity without ever completely abating. His prior workups included hospitalization with CAT scans of the brain and a lumbar puncture.

He reported a distinct improvement after being tested with the mold extracts and receiving his first therapeutic injection. The second injection a few days later cleared all symptoms for the first time since the onset 2 years previously. His symptoms now recur every fourth day and disappear within 30 minutes after an injection. He remains clear as long as he obtains his injection twice a week. Double-blind placebo substitution for his injections causes symptoms to recur.

Case 6—M.E. was a 68-year-old orthopedic surgeon. He had experienced cardiac arrhythmia accompanied by diarrhea and weakness over the previous months. The weakness had become incapacitating to the point where he feared walking across a room. After one week of mold injections he described himself as 80% better than he had felt in the preceding 10 years, and has continued that way on immunotherapy. He also had a history of anosmia for 30 years, thought to be secondary to chronic atopic sinusitis and recurrent polypectomies. His sense of smell returned after injections began.

Case 7—R.S. was a 36-year-old severely asthmatic woman who worked in a family-owned bakery. Wheat RAST was strongly positive. IgE was 70 I.U. Cultures from her bedroom yielded 16 colonies of *Sporobolomyces*, 1 of *Fusarium*, 48 of bacteria, 2 of yeasts, and 1 of sterile fungus. The bakery yielded 1 of *Penicillium*, 1 of *Rhodotorula*, 5 of *Sporobolomyces*, and 3 of bacteria. After two months on immunotherapy her asthma cleared. She was able to stop all medication and she has continued to work in the bakery.

Case 8—S.K. was a 57-year-old carpenter who became cyanotic merely from walking across the room. He was maximally medicated for asthma and was on oral steroids as well. Pulmonary specialists had hospitalized him for a bronchoscopy and bronchograms and his prognosis was guarded. His IgE was 5,666 I.U. With appropriate immunotherapy he began to improve. His cyanosis disappeared and his exercise tolerance increased. After one year on immunotherapy his IgE was 2,146, he no longer needed steroids and had dropped many of his medications. After two years his IgE had fallen to 1,370 I.U. and he only needed albuterol occasionally.

Case 9—M.D. was a 30-year-old housewife with five years of chronic total body pruritis, headache, and rhinitis. All her symptoms cleared within two months of injections and diet.

Case 10—K.L. was a 41-year-old housewife with a seven month history of giant urticaria. She incidentally had had headaches for 20 years and a perennial rhinitis. On appropriate immunotherapy, all symptoms cleared in less than two months and recurred if injections were late.

Discussion

The above case histories are representative of many successfully treated patients. The findings suggest a treatment method for a variety of allergic disorders which have failed to respond to other forms of treatment. The indications of the specificity and appropriateness of immunotherapy with fungal antigens was reinforced by the use of double-blind placebos and the serendipitous failures of patients who were unable to maintain what proved to be critical restrictive diets.

These cases of resistant asthma, eczema, acne, pruritic dermatoses, weakness, migraine, dizziness, and hyperactivity also represent the basic target organs we observed to be affected. Most patients also complained of perennial allergic rhinitis or sinusitis, but that was secondary to their major complaint. This symptom also cleared when the major complaint cleared.

In these as well as hundreds of other similarly treated cases, the brain was a target organ. Hyperactivity, severe headaches, and non-vertiginous dizziness were the major symptoms in many, and were usually accompanied by profound weakness and/or exhaustion. This program brought dramatic relief to many of these patients. These patients reverted to pre-treatment status with double-blind substitution of placebo injections or dietary indiscretions.

Ambient fungi and commonly ingested foods may cause symptoms in a variety of target organs not customarily thought to be affected in atopic diseases. When the top tolerated dose is determined by intradermal testing and frequently ingested foods are eliminated, dramatic responses occurred. Eventually patients added back foods a day to identify those that triggered symptoms. The offending foods were unique for each case, although the commonest offenders were the ferment foods, meaning those derived from yeasts (breads, cheeses, alcohols, vinegars, processed foods). This is not surprising since processed foods are high in fungal antigens. Many preservatives, enzymes, vitamins, pigments, stabilizers, and flavorings are derived from the fermentation process (1). It is possible that cross-antigenic stimulation is at work.

The techniques described here provide one more tool with which the allergist can demonstrate the impact of the environment on a sensitized individual. Appropriate treatment terminates the adverse effects caused by the interplay between man and his environment.

Recommendations for environmental control

Testing and treating for sensitivity to indoor fungi can clear recalcitrant conditions. Methods for reducing the prevalence of fungi also need to be developed.

In this study over 500 mold plates were exposed in bedrooms before and after a variety of environmental controls. Although these have not yet been subjected to statistical analysis, it is evident that washing the entire room with a borax solution, removing carpet, and closing off forced air ducts reduced ambient fungi.

Because there was such wide variability in patient home location and construction as well as financial resources, a number of different modalities were evaluated in terms of effectiveness in lowering fungi levels.

Simply cleaning all surfaces thoroughly and removing carpet and unnecessary clutter reduced fungi in many bedrooms.

One inexpensive and labor-saving method was to seal the rooms and allow evaporation for 48 hours from an open bowl of one cup of vinegar and one cup of chlorine bleach. Occupants were allowed back into the area 48 hours after removing the mixture. In some cases no improvement was seen, but in over 50%, there was significant reduction in colony counts.

In one case use of the mixture for 48 hours in a bedroom reduced the *Penicillium* colony count from 26 to 2 and the *Sporobolomyces* count from 14 to 1.

Prior to the use of the mix, cultures in the bedroom of a patient with chronic sinusitis yielded 12 colonies of *Cladosporium*, 84 of bacteria, 5 of *Alternaria*, 5 of *Rhodotorula*, and 3 of sterile fungi. After using the mixture, no organisms could be grown on the gravity plates.

More beneficial was the use of a single-room electrostatic precipitator. Mold plates indicated that one week of 24-hour operation reduced ambient fungi by 50-100%.

Although most fungi fall within the size range of one micron to 400 microns, the average size of fungi identified on the plates is around 10 microns. With *Cladosporium*, the commonest mold, one species (*C. sphaerospermum*) has a 3-4.5 micron diameter, another (*C. herbarum*) measures 8-15 by 4-6 microns, while other species can be up to 60 microns long. The electrostatic precipitator we recommended had a capacity of 255 cfm and precipitated particles down to 0.1 micron size (11-13).

Most dramatic of all, however, was the use of ultraviolet fluorescent lights. Placement of these in 8-foot ceilings prevented all fungal growth after two weeks. Further studies are being done to determine optimal spacing of these lights.

One disadvantage of this procedure is that the lights must be wired so they are turned off when animals or people enter the room, since eye damage can result within minutes of exposure. They are not as unobtrusive as a single air pollution control device, but they may be useful for particularly moldy environments such as basements.

Increased ventilation is an important way to reduce

indoor chemical air pollution, but our study showed that increasing ventilation by opening windows increased levels of fungi regardless of which control method was used. Hence, heat exchangers should be used and incoming air should be filtered rather than forgo ventilation.

Most of our efforts were aimed at reducing fungi in bedrooms, since we were attempting to create a hypoallergenic oasis for the patient for at least one-third of the day. Extension of some of these methods to the rest of the home or to business environments would be difficult and/or costly and would clearly require the help of a heating, ventilation and air conditioning (HVAC) engineer.

Hopefully, collaborative efforts between the specialist in environmental medicine and the HVAC engineer would prove synergistically beneficial and prevent others from becoming sensitized to ambient fungi.

References

1. Beuchat LR. *Food and Beverage Mycology.* Westport, CT:AVI Publ., 1978.

2 Lehrer SB, Aukrust L, Salvaggio JE. Respiratory allergy induced by fungi, in Symposium on Immune Factors in Pulmonary Disease. *Clinics in Chest Medicine* 4:23-41, 1983.

3. Holst PE et al. Asthma and fungi in the home.

New Zealand Med J 96:718-20, 1983.

4. Mazar A, Baum GC, Segal E et al. Antibodies to inhalant fungal antigens in patients with asthma in Israel. *Ann Allergy* 47 (5 Part I):361-364, 1981

5. Salvaggio JE, Aukrust L. Mold-induced asthma. *Allergy Clin Immunol* 68:327-46, 1981.

- 6. Terracina F, Rogers SA. In-home fungal studies. *Ann Allergy* 49:1;35-37,1982.

7. Rogers SA. A comparison of commercially available mold survey services. *Ann Allergy* 50:37-43, 1983.

8. Rogers SA. A thirteen-month assessment of local work-leisure-sleep fungal environments. *Ann Allergy* 52:338-41, 1984.

9. Willoughby JW. Diagnosis of allergy by serial dilution end-point titration. *Continuing education for the family physician* 11:3, 1979.

10. Rogers SA. Diagnosing the tight building syndrome. *Env Health Persp* 76: 195-198, 1987.

11. Ellis MB. *Dematiaceous Hyphomycetes.* London: Commonwealth Mycological Inst., 1971.

12. Querholts LO. *The Polyporaceae of the United States, Alaska, and Canada.* Ann Arbor: University of Michigan Press, 1983.

13. Lincoff GH. *The Audubon Society Field Guide to North American Mushrooms.* New York: A.A. Knopf, 1981.

A COMPARISON OF COMMERCIALLY AVAILABLE MOLD SURVEY SERVICES

SHERRY A. ROGERS, M.D., F.A.C.A.

Plates from the County Laboratory, Hollister-Stier and our lab were simultaneously placed in the same locations. Comparisons show increased yield comes from a combination of the latter two and the greatest over-all yield came from our lab. Also multiple-placed plates in the same room show the flora is not static.

IN A PREVIOUS STUDY we found several modifications of mycologic techniques to increase the yield in our home fungal studies.[1] In the present study we were interested in with yet another commercially available service. Some of their plates were saved to assess the effects of shipment on culture results.

Because we had no known standard with which to compare the results, and because we were suspicious that even in the home the fungal flora was not a static phenomenon, we performed an additional study. In this we looked at several plates placed at different heights and locations within the same room. This arrangement was repeated several times in the same room at three different locations within a 24-hour period. This latter study was with our plates only.

Methods

This first study, completed in one day, was conducted in three suburban homes in opposite ends of the city. The resident of each house placed plates in the kitchen, bedroom, family room, basement and outdoors (June). At least three plates were placed in each location. These were a malt agar plate from our laboratory, a Sabouraud dextrose from the County Laboratory and a Rose-Bengal agar from the Hollister-Stier Laboratory. (The latter plate marked "outdoors" does not contain the Rose Bengal ingredient as the four indoor plates do.) The County plates were all exposed for 10-min periods. Ours and those of Hollister Stier were exposed one-half hour outdoors and one hour indoors. They were all exposed according to each laboratory's instructions and taped shut. The County's were returned to their laboratory and Hollister-Stier's were mailed to them. We also kept some

Doctor Rogers is in Private Practice Allergy and is Attending Physician, Community General Hospital, Syracuse, New York.

County and Hollister-Stier plates to read ourselves. Our plates were processed as described in our preceding paper.[1] Great care was taken to open the lid only far enough to obtain a sample of the mold being identified under sterile conditions.

Because the County Laboratory plates and those of Hollister-Stier were transported greater distances than ours (the former by Courrier Service, the latter by the U.S. Postal Service), there was a chance that showering of spores would occur with rough handling. Therefore no attempt at quantitation was made.

Results

When all the plates were read the data were tabulated as follows. The total individual genera obtained in each house were listed individually for each house. No quantitation of each organism was attempted. The results of this experiment are shown in Table I.

Our plates of malt agar had a larger number of genera than did Hollister-Stier or County Lab plates. No new genera were found on the County Lab plates. Also, several molds which we found were not reported by them. In the previous paper we gave many reasons for this.[1] Hollister-Stier reported fewer fungi than we did but more than the County. However, they also reported some fungi which our plates did not produce.

Second, for a few randomly selected rooms we set out duplicate County and Hollister-Stier plates, keeping one set to read for ourselves while returning the other set for the official report as stated above. The comparative results are shown in Table II.

The County Laboratory did not report as many genera of fungi as the plates read by our mycologist but we retained the plates for a few weeks to give the slow growers a chance to form colonies.

Although Penicillium was not detected on our plates or on those reported by Hollister-Stier, we did detect a

Table 1. For Each of Three Houses, Five of Our Malt Agar Plates, Five Sabouraud Agar Plates From The County Lab (Co) and Five Of Rose-Bengal Agar (H.S.) Were Exposed. Fungi Reported From Each Of The Three Labs Are Tabulated. At The Asterix H.S. Actually Reported Polyporus (A Basidiomycete).

	FM's house			SG's house			CF's house		
	Ours	Co	HS	Ours	Co	HS	Ours	Co	HS
Cladosporium	+	+		+	+	+	+	+	+
Penicillium	+	+	+		+	+	+	+	+
Sterile		+			+	+	+	+	+
Basidiomycetes	+	+	+*	+	+	+	+		
Alternaria	+			+	+		+		+
Aureobasidium				+			+		+
Epicoccum	+			+			+		
Yeast				+			+		
Paecilomyces	+					+			+
Aspergillus									+
Bacteria				+					
Geotrichum								+	
Rhodotorula								+	
Mortierella	+								
Rhizopus				+					
Curvularia				+					
Sphaeriodaceae				+					
Trichoderma							+		
Botrytis							+		
Fusarium									+
Stemphylium									+

Table II. In The Bedroom of CF's House, One of Our Malt Agar Plates, Two Sabouraud Agar Plates (Co) and Two Rose-Bengal Plates (H.S.) Were Exposed. We Saved One of Each To Read Ourselves and Compare With The Commercial Reading.

	Our malt*	County-SD They read	County-SD We read	HS-Rose Bengal They read	HS-Rose Bengal We read
Cladosporium	+	+	+	+	+
Alternaria	+	+		+	+
Basidiomycetes	+	+			+
Penicillium			+	+	
Fusarium				+	+
Epicoccum	+		+		
Sterile	+	+			
Botrytis			+		+
Aureobasidium	+				
Yeast			+		
Bacteria			+		

Basidiomycete and Botrytis which were not detected by Hollister-Stier plates. This divergence led us to perform the last part of the experiment.

Mold surveys using malt agar only were conducted 11 months later in one room of two houses studied. Simultaneously three plates were exposed in each room at varying heights and locations within the room. In addition, additional malt agar plates were exposed in the same locations every six to 12 hours for a total of 24 hours. The results of this study are given in Tables IIIa and IIIb. As can be seen in Table IIIa, multiple plates exposed in the same room at the same time did not demonstrate the same fungi. Also, at 6:00 p.m. during the period when air turbulence is at its maximum due to human traffic, more fungi were detected on the plates. Samples at high locations (e.g., refrigerator top) revealed fewer molds than samples at low locations such as countertops and floors. Minimum levels of molds were found at midnight. In the second household, similar quantitative results were obtained with regard to numbers of mold.

Discussion

A knowledge of the ambient fungal flora is important to the management of allergic patients.[3] However, all methods of sampling have some degree of inefficiency.[2] First, there is no perfect sampling device. Although gravity plates are easily manageable and economical, only viable numbers of spore are detected. Moreover, viability does not necessarily equate with antigenicity. Many factors other than the presence of spores influence fall-out into the plate. These include room air currents as well as the physical characteristics of the spores, such as size and density, also static spore traps have a layer of dead air space over their surfaces, tending to minimize spore fall-out.[4]

Suction devices and moving impactors are often expensive, clumsy to use for patient home sampling, collect debris other than mold spores, often necessitate spore identification (which is more difficult than identification from a growing colony) and tend to by-pass the smaller spores.[5]

Moreover, there is no optimal medium on which to grow these fungi. Malt agar and Sabouraud dextrose agar plates have been reported to be superior to Rose Bengal,[6] a finding we cannot substantiate in our small study. The antibiotic in Rose Bengal inhibits the growth of some fungi entirely. None of these media support many of the Basidiomycetes such as the rusts and smuts.

Some studies have attempted a variety of methods[7] and indeed at this point it is probably best to persist in individualizing the needs of each allergic patient.[8]

Not only does the amount of physical activity in the environment increase the yield, as we and others[9] have seen, but also affects the number of genera.

Table IIIa. Our Malt Agar Plates Were Exposed at Three Different Locations Within the Same Room of SG's House, Every Six Hours for 24 Hours. The Molds Recovered Are Shown.

	6:00 a.m.			12 noon			6:00 p.m.			12 midnight		
	C	R	F	C	R	F	C	R	F	C	R	F
Cladosporium	+		+	+				+	+	+		+
Sterile	+	+	+			+	+	+	+	+		+
Penicillium				+	+	+		+	+		+	+
Aspergillus				+	+						+	+
Aureobasidium	+			+				+	+	+		
Yeast			+	+	+	+	+	+	+			
Bacteria	+			+	+		+	+	+			
Geotrichum	+	+	+							+		
Rhodotorula							+	+	+			
Actinomycetes				+				+	+			
Alternaria								+	+			
Phoma							+	+				
Basidiomycetes			+							+		
Epicoccum			+									

C—Kitchen counter
R—Top of refrigerator
F—Floor

Table IIIb. Our Malt Agar Plates Were Exposed at Three Different Locations Within the Same Room of CF's House, Three Times Within 24 Hours. The Molds Recovered Are Shown.

	6:00 a.m.			6:00 p.m.			12 midnight		
	F	T	D	F	T	D	F	T	D
Penicillium	+	+	+	+	+	+	+	+	+
Yeast	+	+		+	+	+	+	+	+
Sterile	+	+	+	+	+	+	+	+	+
Cladosporium	+	+	+	+	+				
Aureobasidium		+	+		+	+		+	+
Geotrichum	+	+	+		+	+	+		+
Aspergillus	+	+		+		+			+
Rhodotorula	+	+							+
Actinomycetes		+		+	+	+			
Bacteria				+	+		+		
Black yeast				+		+	+		
Alternaria	+			+					
Phoma				+			+		
Verticillium							+		
Basidiomycetes	+								
Rhizopus						+			

F—living room, fireplace
T—top of TV
D—floor by door

In our previous study[1] we showed that Sabouraud's media used by the County, employing shorter exposure and incubation times gave a lower yield of fungi. The results of the present study shown in Table I demonstrate the effects of these variables. We next evaluated the effects of the size of the plates and length of transit times in shipping on the yield of organisms. No evidence to substantiate this was obtained. Comparative studies with Rose Bengal and malt agar would determine whether the discrepancy lies in the medium itself. Because Rose Bengal did detect fungi that we did not obtain, there seems to be additional benefit in having a Rose Bengal plate as well. There is, of course, the question of which is preferrable, a malt agar plate and a Rose Bengal plate or several randomly placed malt agar plates at peak activity time, repeated throughout the year.

Conclusion

In this study our malt agar plates detected far more genera of fungi in houses than Hollister-Stier's Rose Bengal plates, which far exceeded those employed by the County Laboratory. Each plate detected individual genera of fungi not detected by the other. No additional fungi were found using the County plates. It appears that a malt agar and Rose Bengal plate should give increased yield. Also, increased yield was observed by exposing plates during the time of peak activity in the home (6:00 p.m.) and having plates at a level of four feet or lower. Multiple plates will decrease the chance of missing some ambient spores.

Summary

Plates from the County Laboratory, Hollister-Stier and our lab were simultaneously placed in the same locations. Comparisons show increased yield comes from a combination of the latter two and the greatest over-all yield came from our lab. Also multiple placed plates in the same room showed variations in flora.

Acknowledgments

I acknowledge with gratitude the preparation and reading of all our plates by Fred Terracina, Ph.D., taxonomic mycologist, at the State University of New York, College of Environmental Science and Forestry.

Also appreciation goes to Kathleen Ascioti for typing of the manuscript.

References

1. Terracina F and Rogers S: In-home fungal studies. Ann Allerg 49: 35, 1982.
2. Solomon WR: In Allergy: Principles and Practice, Middleton E, Reed C and Ellis E (Eds.). St Louis: C. V. Mosby Company, 1978.
3. Chapman JA: The enhancement of the practice of clinical allergy with daily pollen and spore counts. Immunol & Allerg Pract IV: 1, 1982.
4. Mallock D: *Molds: Their Isolation, Cultivation and Identification.* University of Toronto Press, p. 37, 1981.
5. Solomon WR, Burge HA, Boise JR and Beelen M: Comparative particle recoveries by the retracting rotorod, rotoslide and Burkard Spore Trap sampling in a compact array. Int J Biometeor 24, 2: 107–116, 1980.

6. Burge HP, Solomon WR and Boise JR: Comparative merits of eight popular media in aerometric studies of fungi. JACI 60, 3: 199–203, 1977.

7. Kozak P, Gallup J, Cummins LH and Gillmon SA: Ann Allergy 45: 85, 1980.

8. ibid II. Samples of problem homes surveyed. 45: 169, 1980.

9. Burge HP, Boise JR and Solomon WR: Fungi in libraries: an aerometric survey. Myopathologia 64: 2, 67–72, 1978.

Requests for reprints should be addressed to:
Dr. Sherry A. Rogers
280 West Genesee Street
Syracuse, New York 13219

AN EXCHANGE OF NOTES

"... We cannot dedicate, we cannot consecrate, we cannot hallow, this ground. The brave men, living and dead, who struggled here, have consecrated it, far above our poor power to add or to detract ... It is for us, the living, rather, to be dedicated here, to the unfinished work that they have thus far so nobly carried on. It is rather for us to be here dedicated to the great task remaining before us; that from these honored dead we take increased devotion to that cause for which they here gave the last full measure of devotion; that we here highly resolve that these dead shall not have died in vain ..."

From President Lincoln's "remarks" at
the dedication of the National Soldiers'
Cemetery at Gettysburg, November 19, 1863.

"... I would be glad if I could flatter myself that I came as near to the central idea of the occasion in two hours as you did in two minutes ..."

Note from Edward Everett, orator at the
dedication.

"... In our respective parts yesterday, you could not have been excused to make a short address, nor I a long one. I am pleased to know that, in your judgment, the little I did say was not entirely a failure ..."

President Lincoln's reply to Mr. Everett.

IN-HOME FUNGAL STUDIES: METHODS TO INCREASE THE YIELD

FRED TERRACINA, Ph.D., and SHERRY A. ROGERS, M.D., F.A.C.A.

This paper shows that by increasing the exposure time from 10 minutes to one hour, substituting malt agar for Sabouraud's dextrose agar and observing the plates beyond one week for four to six weeks, an increase in the variety of genera was noted, above that previously reported.

Introduction

IN A RECENT STUDY of patients with inhalant allergies the incidence of mold allergy was 86%.[1] Airborne fungi are frequently associated with allergic manifestations.[2] There is a growing armamentarium of commercially available mold extracts. However, over the last decade the reports from our local county laboratory on mold surveys done in our patients' homes and offices generally fell into one of three categories: (1) no growth, (2) Basidiomycetes, (3) one or more of the "four mold" group Cladosporium (Hormodendrum), Alternaria, Penicillium and Aspergillus.

The high frequency of Basidiomycetes and the low frequency of genera other than the basic four molds raised the following questions. The first was whether this survey reflected the genera present. The second was whether the Sabouraud's dextrose agar used by our county laboratory and commonly used in medical laboratories would give different results from malt agar, which is commonly used by non-medical mycologists who generally study airborne fungi. Third, we were also interested in whether longer exposures than the 10 minutes exposure recommended by our county laboratory would yield more genera. The fourth was whether plates incubated longer than four days, which was the incubation time used for the county surveys, would yield other genera.

Therefore we decided to do a small study of 10 plates in each of seven residences within the Syracuse metropolitan area.

Materials and Methods

Sterile, disposable Petri dishes (90 × 15 mm) contain-

Fred Terracina, Ph.D., is a Taxonomic Mycology Research Associate, College of Environmental Science & Forestry, S.U.N.Y., Syracuse, New York.

Doctor Rogers is in the private practice of allergy, Attending Community General Hospital, 2800 W. Genesee Street, Syracuse, New York 13219

ing Sabouraud's dextrose Agar (Difco-B109) or 3% malt extract plus 2.0% agar were exposed for one hour in the following four rooms of seven houses: (1) master bedroom, (2) basement, (3) family room and (4) major bathroom. Another exposure for 15 minutes was done with both media in the family rooms of each home. Descriptive data of each house were taken which summarized site location (i.e., city, suburb, rural), type (ranch, cape, etc.) construction (brick, wood, block), heating method, humidification and insulation type, if any. The presence or absence of stored wood was also noted as well as electrostatic precipitators.

The plates were marked, taped shut and incubated in the dark at 24°C. Each plate was examined at the end of four days and bi-weekly thereafter for four to six weeks. Identifications were made from slides made directly from the exposed plates or from subcultures plated onto the appropriate diagnostic media, depending on the fungus being studied.

Results

The results from 70 plates are tabulated in Tables I and II. The order of listing in both tables is based on decreasing frequency. Nineteen taxa were identified. Eighteen of the taxa (95%) were collected on malt extract agar. Twelve taxa (63%) were collected on Sabouraud's dextrose agar.

Although plates from individual rooms remained sterile, no houses examined were free of fungal growth. Bacteria were present in every house sampled and constituted the second most frequently occurring taxon. Aspergillus was also present in every house sampled. Penicillium was common in five of the seven houses examined. Trichoderma did not become identifiable until well after the first week. Basidiomycetes were found in four of the seven houses. They were also more frequently found on malt agar than Sabouraud's agar.

The populations displayed on the media were rather similar, with the most frequently appearing organisms appearing on both media (11 of the 19 taxa involved). Sorenson's Quotient of Similarity[3] was used to estimate the similarity between the two media.

$$Q = \frac{2J}{A + B} \times 100$$

where J = # of taxa in common
A = # of taxa on malt extract agar
B = # of taxa on Sabouraud's dextrose agar

In this analysis identical communities would have a Q of 100. Our results yielded a Q of 80.

Table I. Comparison of Rates of Recovery of Fungi Utilizing Two Different Culture Media

Taxa	Malt agar (%)	Sabouraud dextrose agar (%)
Cladosporium spp.	57	34
Bacteria	43	46
Aspergillus spp.	29	26
Penicillium spp.	23	26
Yeasts (other than Rhodotorula)	29	17
Basidiomycetes	26	20
Rhodotorula sp.	14	9
Trichoderma viride Pers ex Fries	14	3
Epicoccum purpurascens Exrenb ex Schlect	3	6
Alternaria alternata (Fr.) Keissler	9	3
Microsphaeriopsis olivacea (Bonord) Hohn	6	6
Aureobasidium pullulans (De Bary) Arnold	6	0
Sterile moniliaceous	0	6
Sterile dematiaceous	6	0
Phialophora heteromorpha (Nannf.) Wang	3	0
Scytalidium lignicola Pesante	3	0
Stachybotrys atra Corda	3	0
Stephanosporium cerealis (Thum.) Swart	3	0
Wallemia sebi (Fr.) v. Arx	3	0

Discussion

Gregory[4] and Hirst[5] summarized many outdoor surveys of airborne fungi. Indoor surveys are not as frequently performed.[6] Lacey[7] presents a concise overview of the aerobiology of conidial fungi. Recent trends in residential energy conservation (retrofitting) include reducing air infiltration of existing homes, replacing air conditioners with large ceiling circulating fans, increasing humidity and placing insulating materials within the exterior walls that, under elevated moisture conditions, support the growth of many fungi. These considerations, then, may lead to increased numbers of kinds of fungi within the living spaces, particularly during the long winter months in the north temperate zone. Our study was not large enough to draw clear conclusions in this area.

We recognize that our listing of taxa contains elements at various classification ranks and, therefore, our frequency levels are not strictly comparable because unequal numbers of species are represented in several taxa. Nevertheless, this practice is common with almost all other published studies in this area[8,9,10] and therefore our results may be compared with other workers'.

In our study the genus Cladosporium (Hormodendrum) was isolated more frequently than any other taxon. This is consistent with Lumpkins et al[6] as well as Hirsch & Sossman[9] and many previous studies of outdoor samples.[7] Within this taxon three different species were collected: C. cladosporoides, Fresen (deVries), C. herbarium Link ex Fr. and C. sphaerospermum Penzig.

Examples of the genus Aspergillus recovered included Aspergillus flavus group (resembling A. flavus Link var. columnaris Rapar and Fennell), Aspergillus fumigatus Fresenius, Aspergillus niger V. Tiegh and Aspergillus clavatus Desm.

The most frequent Penicillia isolated in our study were Penicillium notatum Westling and Penicillium thomii Maire. The frequency of the genus Trichoderma in this

Table II. Frequency of Isolation of Fungi from Individual Patient Residences

														Patient
A		B		C		D		E		F		G		
SD*	M**	SD	M	SD	M	SD	M	SD	M	SD	M	SD	M	
+	+	+	+	−	+	+	+	+	+	−	+	+	+	Cladosporium spp.
+	+	+	+	+	+	+	+	−	+	+	+	+	+	Bacteria
−	+	+	+	+	+	−	+	+	+	+	+	−	+	Aspergillus spp.
−	+	−	−	−	+	+	+	+	+	+	−	+	+	Yeasts (other than Rhodotorula)
−	+	−	−	+	+	−	−	+	+	−	−	−	+	Basidiomycetes
−	+	−	−	−	+	+	+	+	+	−	+	+	+	Rhodotorula msp.
−	−	−	−	−	−	−	−	+	+	+	+	−	−	Trichoderma viride
−	−	−	−	+	+	+	−	−	+	−	−	−	−	Epicoccum purpurascens
−	−	−	−	−	+	+	+	−	+	−	−	−	−	Alternaria alternata
−	−	−	+	−	−	−	−	−	−	+	−	−	−	Microsphaeriopsis olivacea
−	−	−	+	−	−	−	−	+	−	−	−	−	−	Aureobasidium pullulans
+	−	−	−	−	−	−	−	−	−	−	−	−	−	Sterile Moniliaceous
−	+	−	−	−	−	−	−	−	−	+	−	−	−	Sterile Dematiaceous
−	−	+	−	−	−	−	−	−	−	−	−	−	−	Phialophora hetoromorpha
−	−	−	−	−	−	+	−	−	−	−	−	−	−	Scytalidium lignicola
−	−	−	−	−	−	+	−	−	−	−	−	−	−	Stachybotrys altra
−	−	−	−	−	−	−	−	+	−	−	−	−	−	Stephanosporium cerealis
+	−	−	−	−	−	−	−	−	−	−	−	−	−	Wallemia sebi

* SD = Sabouraud dextrose agar.
** M = malt agar.

study is higher than one usually finds in the literature.[7] It may be reported as a sterile fungus if plates are discarded prematurely.

No attempt was made to identify the yeasts other than to confirm that the pink yeasts recovered were in the genus Rhodotorula rather than Sporobolomyces.

Several kinds of Basidiomycetes were found but we were not able to identify them using either Nobles[11] or Stalpers[12] keys. Frequent oidia and small clamps were invariably found in those cultures we designated as Basidiomycetes. We suspect that identification of Basidiomycetes to the generic level (e.g., Polyporus and Fomes) can not be accomplished except for laboratories having large collections of referenced cultures available for matings, which is often required for identification at the generic and specific levels. Four of the seven houses we examined yielded Basidiomycetes. This result may indicate that they are more frequent than commonly thought because of changing environmental conditions or that they are missed by other investigators who commonly discard plates before two weeks. They are frequently associated with decaying wood.

Neither medium collected all the taxa recovered but the malt extract agar seemed to have a broader spectrum than the Sabouraud's dextrose agar. No Actinomycetes were found and this may be due to the types of media used.

The frequency of appearance of molds on gravity plates does not allow quantitative estimates of the numbers of fungi present per unit volume. However, it is apparent that the qualitative data they provide when ranked by frequency of appearance of taxons closely mimics the rank order found when quantitative viable methods are used.[13,14] It is likely that the numbers of conidia per unit volume of air exhibits short-term periodic fluctuations depending upon biological fluxes and external environmental factors. We are not convinced that the added expense and inconveniences associated with quantitative collection devices warrants their use for routine investigations of patients' residences.

The high incidence of yeasts, Rhodotorula in particular, and Basidiomycetes bears acknowledgement and further study.

Additional findings worth noting are that the top seven isolates from our 70 plates in order of prevalence were Cladosporium (Hormodendrum), bacteria, Aspergillus, Penicillium, yeasts (other than Rhodotorula), Basidiomycetes and Rhodotorula.

In summary, the results of the present studies indicated the following. (1) There were indeed no houses with no growth. Also there were many more genera present than Basidiomycetes and the basic four molds. (2) Malt extract agar yielded 95% of the fungi, while Sabouraud's dextrose agar yielded 63%. This suggests that the malt extract agar has a better retrieval rate. (3) No plates were overgrown by bacteria to an extent where they interfered with the identification of fungi. (4) Many of the genera were not identifiable during the first week, thus plates should be observed longer.

Therefore, by increasing exposure time from 10 minutes to one hour, substituting malt agar for Sabouraud's dextrose agar and, rather than discarding plates prior to one week, by examining the plates for four to six weeks, the over-all number of genera observed was increased by 32%.

References

1. Speer F, Denison TR, and Baptist JE: Aspirin allergy. Ann Allerg 46: 123–182, 1981.
2. Hyde HA: Atmospheric pollen and spores in relation to allergy. J Clin Allerg 2: 153–159, 1972.
3. Sorensen T: A method of establishing groups of equal amplitude in plant society based on similarity of species content. K Danske Vidansk Selsk 5: 1–34, 1948.
4. Gregory PH: *Microbiology of the Atmosphere*, Second Edition. Leonard Hill, Aylesbury, 1973.
5. Hirst JM: A trapper's line. Trans Br Mycol Soc 61: 205–213, 1973.
6. Lumpkins E, Corbit SL and Tiedeman GM: Airborne fungi survey. I. Culture-plate survey of the home environment. Ann Allerg 31: 361–370, 1973.
7. Lacey J: The aerobiology of conidial fungi. In *Biology of Conidial Fungi*, Volume 1, Cole GT and Kendrick B (Eds.). New York: Academic Press, 1981, pp. 373–416.
8. Levitan E and Horowitz L: A one-year survey of the airborne molds of Tulsa, Oklahoma. II. Indoor survey. Ann Allerg 41: 25–27, 1978.
9. Hirsch SR and Sossman JA: A one-year survey of mold growth inside twelve homes. Ann Allerg 36: 30–38, 1976.
10. Richards M: Atmospheric mold spores in and out of doors. J Allerg 25: 429–439, 1954.
11. Nobles MK: Identification of cultures of wood inhabiting Hymenomycetes. Can J Bot 43: 1097–1139, 1965.
12. Stalpers JA: Identification of wood-inhabiting aphyllophorales in pure culture. Stud Mycol 1:248, 1978.
13. Burge HP, Boise JR, Rutherford JA and Solomon WA: Comparative recoveries of airborne fungus spores by viable and non-viable modes of volumetric collection. Mycopathologia 61: 27–33, 1977.
14. Kozan PP, Gallup J, Cummins LH and Gilman SA: Currently available methods for home mold surveys. II. Examples of problem homes surveyed. Ann Allerg 45: 167–176, 1980.

Requests for reprints should be addressed to:
Dr. Sherry A. Rogers
2800 W. Genesee Street
Syracuse, New York 13219

A 13-MONTH WORK-LEISURE-SLEEP ENVIRONMENT FUNGAL SURVEY

SHERRY A. ROGERS, M.D., F.A.C.A

Thirty plates per month for 13 months were exposed in patients' work-leisure-sleep environments in central New York State. Results show the months of highest mold prevalence in decreasing order were October, September, May and July. These months are also typically our high pollen months.

The categories of highest prevalence in decreasing order were yeasts, mycelia sterilia, Cladosporium, Penicillium, Rhodotorula, bacteria, Alternaria, Aureobasidium, Epicoccum, Aspergillus, Geotrichum, Basidiomycetes, Actinomycetes and Phoma. These were present in at least 14% of all 390 plates.

The present study includes a discussion of the value of these findings in an allergy practice.

Introduction

PREVIOUSLY WE PRESENTED a method to increase the yield of fungi isolated in our in-home fungal studies.[1,2] We found a different media, a longer exposure time and a longer reading time gave increased yields. In the light of these findings the purpose of the present study was to assess the fungal environment in our area over a period of 13 months. Surveys were done of work-leisure-sleep areas to obtain data that would more nearly reflect a patient's 24-hour exposure.

Materials and Methods

One-hundred and thirty allergy patients were randomly selected from an allergy practice. Each month for 13 months (June, 1981, to June, 1982), 10 different patients exposed three plates each in their environments.

For all patients culture plates were exposed in the bedroom. For the second plate most chose the family room or basement, depending upon where they spent leisure time. The third plate was exposed at the place of employment which was often an office, home kitchen, barn or outdoors. Thus we attempted to obtain a representation of the fungal exposures for a person who has three major areas of exposure: work-leisure-

Presented at the 39th Annual Congress of the American College of Allergists, January 29–February 2, 1983, New Orleans, Louisianna.
Dr. Rogers is in private practice in allergy and is Attending Physician at Community General Hospital, Syracuse, N.Y.

sleep. All people lived within a 100-mile radius of the city of Syracuse, New York. The plates contained 3% malt extract plus 2.0% agar and were exposed for one hour. Plates were marked, taped shut and stored at room temperature. They were examined twice a week, semi-permanent slides in lactophenol were made and taxa were identified from slides until new colonies ceased to appear, usually two to three weeks.

Results

The data from 390 plates, 30 each month for 13 months, were tabulated. Table I shows the genera of fungi isolated or other taxonomic groups that were identified within the limits of practicality. They are arranged in decreasing order of prevalence based on the percentage of plates from which each was isolated. One hundred percent would mean that taxon was present on all 390 plates.

Figure 1 is a bar graph illustrating the 14 most prevalent taxa. These were also present in at least 14% of the 390 plates.

The six most divergent months from the 13-month average were February, March, May, July, September and October. February and March had far fewer fungi isolated than all the other months. May, July, September and October were the months of highest mold prevalence, well above the average for the year. For each taxon, the order from top to bottom in the bar graphs is May, July, September, October 1 to the 13-month average.

Some of the recent changes in fungal taxonomy

Table I. Percentage of Plates on Which Present (Total 390 Plates).

1.	Yeasts	78%	11.	Geotrichum	16%
2.	Mycelia sterilia	65	12.	Basidiomycetes	16
3.	Cladosporium	63	13.	Actinomycetes	16
4.	Penicillium	52	14.	Phoma	14
5.	Rhodotorula	45	15.	Dematiaceous fungi	8
6.	Bacteria	44	16.	Fusarium	6
7.	Alternaria	44	17.	Rhizopus	5
8.	Aureobasidium	40	18.	Trichoderma	5
9.	Epicoccum	23	19.	Paecilomyces	3
10.	Aspergillus	23	20.	Beauveria	3

Present on 1% of plates

Monocillium	pycnidial-producing (non-Phoma)
Stachybotrys	Acremonium
Arthrinium	Botrytis
Scopulariopsis	Candida
Gilmaniella	Ulocladium
Zygomycetes	

Only one colony each

Monodictys	Graphium
Helminthosporium	Crysosporium
Sepadonium	Thysanophora
Oidiodendron	Nigrospora
sclerotial-producing	Gliomastix
Custingophora	

include *Cladosporium* (*Hormodendrum*), *Aureobasidium* (*Pullularia*) and *Acremonium* (*Cephalosporium*).

Discussion

September is not only the height of the ragweed season but also the month of second highest airborne fungal prevalence. The results of published studies suggest that in some patients we may be identifying the wrong etiologic allergen, at least underestimating the total antigenic load.

During the month of October the largest number of fungi were recovered. This may in part account for the "persistence of symptoms" after the ragweed season (i.e., the first October frost). Lopez et al and Santilli et al have suggested that the basidiomycetes may be in part responsible for fall symptoms.

The yeasts were the predominant category identified each month. How antigenic these and other categories are remains to be elucidated. Moreover, the complete identification of yeasts is beyond the expertise of most allergists. Possibly a large percentage is represented by only a few of the many genera of yeasts that exist.

The yeast *Rhodotorula* is distinguished by its glistening pink globular colonies and therefore was categorized separately. Adding *Rhodotorula*, the fifth most prevalent category, to the yeast category, which is the number one most prevalent category each month, makes this taxon even more assuming. Candida is also a yeast but can be identified to genus by its white to cream-colored yeast-like colonies at 25 C° and the presence of pseudomycelia.

The bacteria, number 6 in prevalence and present in 50% of the cultures, were also not further differentiated

since these require diagnostic media and techniques not employed in the present studies.

Aureobasidium (*Pullularia*) is number 8 in prevalence. Our area has many transient people who upon transfer here enable us to see previous allergy records from all over the country. This genera is not frequently tested.

The basidiomycetes were identified only if a clamp connection was seen. Some of the mycelia sterilia may have been basidiomycetes as well. In other laboratories many plates may be discarded before the laborious task of seeking clamp connections has been undertaken, leaving them to be added to the mycelia sterilia category. This may be an important observation since mycelia sterilia constitute the second most common classification. Basidiomycetes do not lend themselves easily to further differentiation in culture and rusts and smuts would not be expected to be detected on this medium, since they are basidiomycetes which are strict plant pathogens. Many deuteromycetes are pleomorphic, in that in spite of possessing one genotype, they can produce two or more phenotypes. This may be dependent upon availability of nutrients. This leads to the speculation among taxonomic mycologists that many deuteromycetes (and this includes yeasts) represent the asexual phase of organisms that really belong to the class basidiomycetes.[5a]

The actinomycetes, a group of organisms closely related to bacteria (pro-karyotes), were a surprising observation since our media and methods were not ideal for the isolation of these organisms.[6]

This category might be more prevalent if studies were to be done under conditions appropriate for their growth.

In addition to basidiomycetes, the mycelia sterilia may represent imperfect fungi. Again, many of these fungi may have nutrient requirements not provided for in the present studies. The inclusion of petri dishes containing other media in a survey may help further identifications of unsuspected fungi.[2,5b]

The pycnidial-producing organisms included all the Sphaeropsidales except *Phoma*, which is easy to identify by its characteristic large black pycnidium.[7]

Some of the dematiaceous fungi could have been included in the mycelia sterilia, making it even more expansive, but were easily separated due to their dark mycelia. The categories were not all at the same taxonomic level but identification was taken as far as was practical.

Because *Rhodotorula*, *Aureobasidium*, *Epicoccum* and *Geotrichum* are fungi that are commonly isolated but infrequently tested for, it may be worthwhile testing patient reactions to extracts of these in addition to the four that are commonly tested for (*Cladosporium*, *Penicillium*, *Alternaria*, *Aspergillus*). Perhaps other fungi should be tested for antigenic importance if they are significant in the patient's 24-hour exposure.

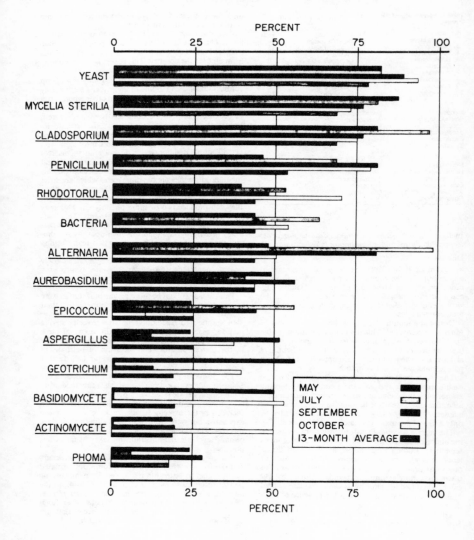

Conclusion

In view of the improvement in our techniques and lack of recent local surveys, a 13-month survey was done to assess the local work-leisure-sleep environments. The times of highest fungal prevalence occurred concurrently with the highest pollen seasons and worst seasons, symptom-wise, for many patients. Yeasts and bacteria have high prevalence but are not commonly tested for reactivity in allergic individuals. Basidiomycetes and actinomycetes were also prevalent. All four of these taxonomic groups require sophisticated studies to further identify their members. Additional studies may also be required to see if antigenicity exists for type 1 atopy.

Rhodotorula, Aureobasidium, Epicoccum, Geotrichum and *Phoma* seem to merit placement in intradermal test sets along with the four commonly tested major fungi (*Cladosporium, Penicillium, Alternaria* and *Aspergillus*). Other fungi could be tested depending upon the results of patients' individual 24-hour environmental culture results.

Acknowledgments

The author is grateful for the reading of all plates by Mr. Chin Shan Yang, word-processing by Mrs. Bonnie

Worden and the generous technical advise of Dr. Fred Terracina, taxonomic mycologist, and illustrative services of Mr. Doug Whitman.

References

1. Terracina F., Rogers, SA.: In-home fungal studies: methods to increase the yield. Ann Allergy 49: 35–37, 1982.
2. Rogers, SA.: A comparison of commercially available mold survey services. Ann Allergy 50, #1: 37–40, 1983.
3. Lopez, M., Salvaggio, J. and Butcher, B.: Allergenicity and immunogenicity of basidiomycetes. JACI 57 #5: 480–488, 1976.
4. Santilli, J., March, DG., Collins, RP, Alexander, JF. and Norman, PS.: Basidiospore sensitivity and asthma. JACI 69, #1, Part 2: p. 98. 1982.
5a. Al-Doory Y. and Domson F.: *Mould Allergy.* Lea & Febiger, Philadelphia, chapter 2, 1984.
5b. Ibid, chapter 3.
6. *Fungi of Pulp & Paper in New York,* Wang, CJK. Technical Publication #87. State Univ. College of Forestry at Syracuse Univ., p. 92–95, 1965.
7. *Illustrated Genera of Imperfect Fungi,* Barnett, HL., and Hunter, DB. Burgess Publ. Co., Minneapolis, Minnesota 1972.

Requests for reprints should be addressed to:
Doctor Sherry A. Rogers
2800 West Genesee Street
Syracuse, New York 13219

Advice for the Physician

"Sometimes give your services for nothing, calling to mind a previous benefaction or present satisfaction. And if there by an opportunity of serving one who is a stranger in financial straits, give full assistance to all such. For where there is love of man, there is also love of the art. For some patient, though conscious that their condition is perilous, recover their health simply through their contentment with the goodness of the physician. And it is well to superintend the sick to make them well, to care for the healthy to keep them well, also to care for one's self, so as to observe what is seemly."

Hippocrates

THE E. I. SYNDROME

"ARE YOU ALLERGIC TO THE 21st CENTURY?"
AN RX FOR ENVIRONMENTAL ILLNESS

By Sherry A. Rogers, M. D.

HERE'S THE BOOK YOU'VE BEEN WAITING FOR
A MUST FOR EVERY E.I. PATIENT AND DOCTOR

Dr. Sherry Rogers teaches in the Advanced Course for Physicians learning Environmental Medicine, and has lectured throughout China with Dr.'s Randolph and Rea, as well as in Canada, England and through- out the United States. She has published studies on mold allergy, as well as the provocation-neutralization testing for chemical sensitiv- ities. She has written articles in many health magazines and news- letters on every aspect of Environmental Illness.

This 600 page manual for patients is crammed full of pearls and spells out the workup for the most mildly allergic person, right on through to the universal reactors, which Dr. Rogers, herself, is. It goes through everything the patient needs to know about mold and other inhalant allergies, food allergies, chemical allergies, Candida syndrome, nutritional deficiencies, toxicities of xenobiotics, and the psychoneurolimmune connection.

Six years ago the book started out as a few handouts to patients, and every question that was ever asked was recorded so that some- where in these 600 pages, it could be answered. Time and again patients say, "Everytime I read the book I learn something new. There's just so much I couldn't possibly get it all the first or second time."

To order: Send $15 plus $3 postage for each book desired.

NAME: _____

ADDRESS:_____

_____

Enclosed is _____ for _____ copies of The E.I. Syndrome

Send to: Prestige Publishers   Or: Dr. Sherry A. Rogers
            Box 3161   2800 W. Genesee St.
            3500 Brewerton Rd.   Syracuse, N.Y. 13219
            Syracuse, N.Y. 13220